AF870900

OTHER *ESSENTIALS* BOOKS

Essentials on **ADOLESCENT HEALTH FOR NURSING AND HEALTH PROFESSIONALS**: A Care Guide (*Herrman*)

Essentials for the **ADULT-GERONTOLOGY ACUTE CARE NURSE PRACTITIONER** (*Carpenter*)

Essentials for the **ANTEPARTUM AND POSTPARTUM NURSE**: A Nursing Orientation and Care Guide (*Davidson*)

Essentials Workbook for **CARDIAC DYSRHYTHMIAS AND 12-LEAD EKGs** (*Desmarais*)

Essentials for the **CARDIAC SURGERY NURSE**: Caring for Cardiac Surgery Patients, Third Edition (*Hodge*)

Essentials for **CAREER SUCCESS IN NURSING**: Making the Most of Mentoring (*Vance*)

Essentials for the **CATH LAB NURSE**, Second Edition (*McCulloch*)

Essentials for the **CLASSROOM NURSING INSTRUCTOR**: Classroom Teaching (*Yoder-Wise, Kowalski*)

Essentials for the **CLINICAL NURSE LEADER** (*Wilcox, Deerhake*)

Essentials for the **CLINICAL NURSE MANAGER**: Managing a Changing Workplace, Second Edition (*Fry*)

Essentials for the **CLINICAL NURSING INSTRUCTOR**: Clinical Teaching, Third Edition (*Kan, Stabler-Haas*)

Essentials on **COMBATING NURSE BULLYING, INCIVILITY, AND WORKPLACE VIOLENCE**: What Nurses Need to Know (*Ciocco*)

Essentials About **COMPETENCY-BASED EDUCATION IN NURSING**: How to Teach Competency Mastery (*Wittmann-Price, Gittings*)

Essentials for the **CRITICAL CARE NURSE**, Second Edition (*Hewett*)

Essentials About **CURRICULUM DEVELOPMENT IN NURSING**: How to Develop and Evaluate Educational Programs, Second Edition (*McCoy, Anema*)

Essentials for **DEMENTIA CARE**: What Nurses Need to Know, Second Edition (*Miller*)

Essentials for **DEVELOPING A NURSING ACADEMIC PORTFOLIO**: What You Really Need to Know (*Wittmann-Price*)

Essentials About **DIVERSITY, EQUITY, AND INCLUSION IN NURSING**: Building Competencies for an Antiracism Practice (*Davis*)

Essentials for **DNP ROLE DEVELOPMENT**: A Career Navigation Guide (*Menonna-Quinn, Tortorella Genova*)

Essentials About **EKGs FOR NURSES**: The Rules of Identifying EKGs (*Landrum*)

Essentials for the **ER NURSE**: Guide to a Successful Emergency Department Orientation, Fourth Edition (*Buettner*)

Essentials for **EVIDENCE-BASED PRACTICE IN NURSING**: Third Edition (*Godshall*)

Essentials for the **FAITH COMMUNITY NURSE**: Implementing FCN/Parish Nursing (*Hickman*)

Essentials About **FORENSIC NURSING**: What You Need to Know (*Scannell*)

Essentials on **GENETICS AND GENOMICS FOR NURSES**: Practical Applications (*Subasic*)

Essentials for the **GERONTOLOGY NURSE**: A Nursing Care Guide (*Eliopoulos*)

Essentials About **GI AND LIVER DISEASES FOR NURSES**: What APRNs Need to Know (*Chaney*)

Essentials About the **GYNECOLOGICAL EXAM**: A Professional Guide for NPs, PAs, and Midwives, Second Edition (*Secor, Fantasia*)

Essentials in **HEALTH INFORMATICS FOR NURSES** (*Hardy*)

Essentials for **HEALTH PROMOTION IN NURSING**: Promoting Wellness (*Miller*)

Essentials for Nurses About **HOME IN FUSION THERAPY**: The Expert's Best Practice Guide (*Gorski*)

Essentials for the **HOSPICE NURSE**: A Concise Guide to End-of-Life Care, Second Edition (*Wright*)

Essentials about **LGBTQ+ CARE FOR NURSES** (*Traister*)

Essentials for the **LONG-TERM CARE NURSE**: What Nursing Home and Assisted Living Nurses Need to Know (*Eliopoulos*)

Essentials to **LOVING YOUR RESEARCH PROJECT**: A Stress-Free Guide for Novice Researchers in Nursing and Healthcare (*Marshall*)

Essentials for **MAKING THE MOST OF YOUR CAREER IN NURSING** (*Redulla*)

Essentials for **MANAGING PATIENTS WITH APSYCHIATRIC DISORDER**: What RNs, NPs, and New Psych Nurses Need to Know (*Marshall*)

Essentials About **MEDICAL CANNABIS AND OPIOIDS**: Minimizing Opioid Use Through Cannabis (*Smith, Smith*)

Essentials for the **MEDICAL OFFICE NURSE**: What You Really Need to Know (*Richmeier*)

Essentials for the **MEDICAL–SURGICAL NURSE**: Clinical Orientation (*Ciocco*)

Essentials for **MIDWIVES**: Labor & Delivery Orientation, Third Edition (*Groll*)

Essentials for the **OPERATING ROOM NURSE**, Third Edition (*Criscitelli*)

Essentials for **PATIENT SAFETY IN NURSING**: How to Decrease Medical Errors and Improve Patient Outcomes (*Hunt*)

Essentials for **PSYCHOPHARMACOLOGY FOR NURSE PRACTITIONERS** (*Goldin*)

ESSENTIALS for PATIENT SAFETY IN NURSING

Deborah Dolan Hunt, PhD, RN, is Professor Emerita of the College of New Rochelle, Betty L. Forest Dean of Adelphi's College of Nursing and Public Health at Adelphi University, and Fellow of the New York Academy of Medicine. She is thrilled to be publishing this book and has published three prior books with Springer Publishing Company: *The New Nurse Educator: Mastering Academe*, *The Nurse Professional: Leveraging Your Education for Transition into Practice*, and *Essentials About Nursing Practice: Historical Facts in a Nutshell*. She is on the editorial board of DailyNurse.com, serves on the Personalized Medicine Coalition Advisory Panel, and is a guest editor for Frontiers. She is Ambassador and Reviewer with the Patient-Centered Outcomes Research Institute (PCORI) and serves as Co-Chair of the Health and Human Services Committee at Community Board #10, where she spearheaded a healthy lifestyle initiative. She is currently serving as Co-Chair of the Talent Acquisition Committee at the Westchester County Association. She was the principal investigator of the Health Resources and Services Administration (HRSA) grant at College of New Rochelle (CNR) and facilitated its transfer to Mercy College and is currently serving as one of the activity directors for the Title V Access grants. Her research interests are in leadership, patient outcomes, new nurse transition, and mentoring.

Dr. Hunt was Interim Dean at the College of New Rochelle and led the transition of the nursing program to Mercy College. She is an alum of both the College of New Rochelle and Mercy College, which shared a similar mission. Mercy College has welcomed her and the former students, faculty, staff, and administrators with welcoming arms, and she appreciates the collegiality and commitment to service and excellence at all levels.

In addition to academic writing, Dr. Hunt also publishes children's books, and the second edition of her self-care book *Essential Oils, Teas, and Self-Care* will be released in 2022.

ESSENTIALS for PATIENT SAFETY IN NURSING

How to Decrease Medical Errors and Improve Patient Outcomes

Deborah Dolan Hunt, PhD, RN

SPRINGER PUBLISHING

Copyright © 2023 Springer Publishing Company, LLC

All rights reserved.

No part of this publication may be reproduced, stored in a retrieval system, or transmitted in any form or by any means, electronic, mechanical, photocopying, recording, or otherwise, without the prior permission of Springer Publishing Company, LLC, or authorization through payment of the appropriate fees to the Copyright Clearance Center, Inc., 222 Rosewood Drive, Danvers, MA 01923, 978-750-8400, fax 978-646-8600, info@copyright.com or on the Web at www.copyright.com.

Springer Publishing Company, LLC
11 West 42nd Street, New York, NY 10036
www.springerpub.com
connect.springerpub.com/

Acquisitions Editor: Rachel X. Landes
Compositor: Transforma

ISBN: 978-0-8261-8455-9

Printed by LSI

The author and the publisher of this Work have made every effort to use sources believed to be reliable to provide information that is accurate and compatible with the standards generally accepted at the time of publication. Because medical science is continually advancing, our knowledge base continues to expand. Therefore, as new information becomes available, changes in procedures become necessary. We recommend that the reader always consult current research and specific institutional policies before performing any clinical procedure or delivering any medication. The author and publisher shall not be liable for any special, consequential, or exemplary damages resulting, in whole or in part, from the readers' use of, or reliance on, the information contained in this book. The publisher has no responsibility for the persistence or accuracy of URLs for external or third-party Internet websites referred to in this publication and does not guarantee that any content on such websites is, or will remain, accurate or appropriate.

Contact sales@springerpub.com to receive discount rates on bulk purchases.

***Publisher's Note:* New and used products purchased from third-party sellers are not guaranteed for quality, authenticity, or access to any included digital components.**

The *Essentials* series was published in the United States of America as the *Fast Facts* series.

I dedicate this book first and foremost to the patients and their families who have suffered due to a medical error.

To our current and future healthcare professionals who strive every single day to promote positive patient outcomes.

To my children, who inspire me every single day to never give up on my dreams.

To Dr. Jean Watson, who embodies the art and science of nursing and serves as a role model and has had such a profound impact on the nursing profession.

In loving memory of all the individuals who lost their lives due to COVID-19!

In loving memory of Brian Francis Hunt.

Contents

Case Exemplar Contributors

M. Roseann Diehl, PhD, DNP, CRNA, CHSE-A, Professor Professional Practice, Texas Christian University, Harris College of Nursing and Health Sciences, TCU School of Nurse Anesthesia, Fort Worth, Texas

Ashley Mulanax, BSN, RN, CCRN, Nursing Professional Development Generalist, Intensive Care Unit, Confluence Health, Wenatchee, Washington

R. Scott Murphy, Donor Evaluation Coordinator, LiveOnNY, Long Island City, New York

Fermin Renteria, DNP, APRN, CPNP-PC, CNE, Clinical Assistant Professor and Director, BSN Program, University of Arkansas for Medical Sciences College of Nursing, Little Rock, Arkansas

Elizabeth Riley, DNP, PED-BC, RNC-NIC, CNE, Clinical Assistant Professor, College of Nursing, University of Arkansas for Medical Sciences, Little Rock, Arkansas

Christine Rovinski-Wagner, MSN, APRN, Program Manager, Quality Management, Clinical Contact Center Modernization, Office of Veterans Access to Care, Veterans' Health Administration, Washington, District of Columbia

Debra A. Simons, PhD, RN, Dean, School of Nursing and Health Sciences, Manhattanville College, Purchase, New York

Danielle Walker, PhD, RN, CNE, Associate Professor, Harris College of Nursing and Health Professions, Texas Christian University, Fort Worth, Texas

Courtney Wallace, MSN, RN, CPHQ, Nursing Manager, Progressive Care Unit, Central Washington Hospital, Wenatchee, Washington

Foreword

Essentials for Patient Safety in Nursing comes at a special time from a well-established author, Dr. Deborah Hunt, who knows how to engage the readers in using facts, innovation, and informed imagination to revise errors and improve patient SafeCare experiences. The factual content is organized and framed from within, first, from relevant and extant research data, statistics, national support, and major position statements from distinctive scientific-academic boards and organization and then by major professional practice dynamics and demands that need attention to understand and confront/address/overcome adverse events and errors affecting safety.

This text progresses from factual background to and through other dominant dynamics and dimensions that come into play in the entire field of safety. As highlighted throughout, safety and medical nursing errors go hand in hand. These intertwined dynamics require confronting concrete and substantive human-technology core error issues, issues everyone and every hospital knows but somehow continue to haunt institutions and health practitioners.

These intervening safety-error core variables include such basic, common safety deficits as pressure ulcers, falls, and medication errors. They are related to communication, misused technology, workload, staffing education, knowledge, preparation, theory, clinical judgment, prioritization delegation, leadership, and emotional intelligence.

This unique *Essentials* serves as a quick resource text for foundational, relevant data, knowledge, and vital information, not only about the nature of medical errors but also about why they occur. More important, Dr. Hunt shows us how to comprehensively address problems by highlighting the need for both academic and clinical professional development, emphasizing approaches such as theory-informed practices, and acknowledging the importance of human caring, power, relationship, and such practices as "mindful presence."

Chapter 4, "Theory-Informed Practice," is quite comprehensive, indicating how specific theories can improve care and serve as guides to safety and safe practices for yourself and the patient. Some core extant theories are highlighted, such as Barrett's power theory, Watson's Theory of Human Caring, the Relationship-Based Care model, and others, as well as universal concepts of "mindfulness and presence" as core human variables. As noted, these theory-guided professional safety practices cannot occur without education, knowledge, preparation, professional development, basic clinical judgment skills, overall leadership, and other such human dynamics influencing mature safe professional nursing practices.

This book is structured and organized around two major units; each unit has its own evolved pattern and momentum.

Unit I: Adverse Events in Nursing: Identifying the Problem: These are largely human errors but are compounded by institutional practices, workload, technology, professional orientation/education, and other dominant system demands. This unit has two major chapters providing an introduction and overview/context of safety–error concerns.

Unit II: Improving Patient Safety and Decreasing Adverse Events: This unit offers six chapters, taking the reader into more creative solutions and how to "face the facts" through new forms of preparation and informed human action. Special topics identify pending and parallel concerns such as ethics and self-care. The final chapter in Unit II offers a holistic approach, helping all the pieces to fall into place. Here Dr. Hunt provides a synthesis and comprehensive overview of the whole.

Other strengths of this work are quick and user-friendly access to facts through the use of case vignettes, discussion questions, case examplars, and assignments. Summary sections highlight major national safety initiatives with improved outcomes, for example from The Joint Commission, Quality and Safety Education for Nurses, and the National Academy of Medicine, each demonstrating success when national attention is placed on both problems and solutions.

Overall, this work is indeed a *Essentials* resource as well as a fundamental and succinct guide to big-picture, as well as micro and macro, concerns that need to be addressed. It can serve as a most useful resource for any faculty, course, student, practitioner, or administrator. While considered and developed as a *Essentials* text, it is indeed packed, certainly, with not only facts but also comprehensive knowledge and directions for the field. The reference citations alone are a valuable resource for this gem of a book. This factual book is full of the most relevant current and classic reference citations, which will serve well any academician, scholar, educator, and practitioner.

Jean Watson, PHD, RN, AHN-BC, FAAN, LL (AAN)
Founder, Watson Caring Science Institute
Distinguished Professor/Dean Emerita
University of Colorado Denver
Boulder, Colorado

Preface

In 2020, the unthinkable occurred with the emergence of COVID-19 and the pandemic that followed, which caused significant illness and death and changed our way of life in ways we could have never imagined. There was much uncertainty and fear and trial and error. Major interventions included quarantining, masks, and virtually shutting down society to flatten the curve. The development of vaccines and treatments changed the trajectory. Two years later, the number of cases has decreased, but we still live with uncertainty. Every facet of life has been impacted. However, the impact on healthcare, and the resultant shortages across the various disciplines, especially nursing, have been significant. The lessons learned from this unprecedented event should guide future policy and preparedness.

"Do no harm" is a mantra all healthcare professionals embrace. Unfortunately, medical errors and poor quality of care persist despite the stalwart efforts of various healthcare leaders and experts. The purpose of this book is to highlight the alarming statistics regarding medical errors and the most common causes. In 1999 when the landmark report *To Err Is Human: Building a Safer Health Care System* was released, there was a concerted and collaborative effort to change the trajectory and improve patient outcomes by preventing medical errors and adverse outcomes. There were improvements, which are highlighted in this book; however, in recent years, the number of adverse outcomes has increased at an alarming rate. A thorough review of the literature identified the most significant errors and their causes. The significance of critical thinking, logic, and clinical judgment has been well established, and this book includes strategies for developing and improving these skills. The case studies, exemplars, tips from the field, discussion questions, and special topics support the integration and application of the important concepts addressed in this book.

Unit I addresses the severity of the issue and common causes. The first chapter provides an overview of the issue and the agencies that focus on patient safety. Despite numerous policy changes and strategies, patient errors have continued to increase after a previous improvement that stemmed from the initiatives after the publication of *To Err Is Human*. Common medical errors include medication errors, patient falls, pressure ulcers, infections, and surgical errors

The second chapter describes the primary causes with poor communication being one of the most common causes. Other causes include misuse of technology, poorly conceived processes, and workload issues. These types of errors, which occur across healthcare institutions cost approximately $1.7 billion per year and are related to miscommunication, not recording information, ignoring messages, or never receiving them. Other causes include the misuse of technology, poorly conceived processes, and workload issues

Medication errors include failure to properly identify the patient, heavy workloads, staff shortages, noise and distractions, fatigue, sound-alike drugs, the misuse of abbreviations, illegible prescriptions, inappropriate dosage and infusion rates, incorrect time, and poor communication during change of shift. Workload issues have been correlated with poor patient outcomes and the pandemic has certainly exacerbated the nursing and healthcare professional shortage.

Unit II is focused on improving patient safety and decreasing adverse events. The third chapter focuses on ways to become a safe practitioner through education and competency development. The fourth chapter highlights several theories that can be used to promote quality of care and decrease adverse outcomes. The fifth chapter focuses on the significance of critical thinking in promoting patient outcomes and ways to develop and improve critical thinking and reasoning. Clinical judgment is an important skill and Tanner's Clinical Judgment Model has been widely used to help develop clinical judgemnt. The sixth chapter focuses on prioritization and delegation and ways to develop these skills in addition to scope of practice, intuition, and ethics. The seventh chapter focuses on leadership and emotional intelligence, and the final chapter focuses on the issue from a holistic approach and includes cultural humility and artificial intelligence.

Acknowledgments

I signed the contract for this book at a pivotal time in my life; then the pandemic changed our world forever, and I almost didn't get to complete this book. Thanks to Joe Morita and Hannah Hicks from Springer Publishing Company, who encouraged me and patiently waited for me to finish this book, which I hope will play a role in preventing adverse outcomes and promoting patient outcomes and quality of care.

I want to thank and acknowledge all the contributors who generously gave their time and knowledge and who are committed to promoting positive patient outcomes.

I would like to acknowledge the entire team at Springer who helped bring this book to fruition.

And thanks to my dear friend and mentor Dr. Jean Watson for writing the foreword of this book.

I

Adverse Events in Nursing: Identifying the Problem

1

Patient Safety and Adverse Events: The Big Picture

Paper doesn't save people, people save people.
–Dan Petersen, Safety Professional

Patient safety is at the forefront of every healthcare organization. Despite initiatives from organizations such as Quality and Safety Education for Nurses (QSEN), The Joint Commission (TJC), and the Institute of Medicine (IOM), the rates of preventable harm among patients are still too high.

In this chapter you will learn:

1. About key areas in patient safety and adverse events
2. Factors related to medication errors, patient falls, pressure ulcers, and infections
3. How to describe QSEN and the competencies
4. Initiatives by the IOM
5. TJC initiatives on patient safety

BACKGROUND

According to the World Health Organization (WHO; 2019), one out of every four patients receiving primary or ambulatory care is harmed. The IOM estimates that medical errors cost between $17 and $29 billion per year. Domestically, according to a well-publicized 2016 study from Johns Hopkins, medical errors are the third-largest cause of death, with an estimate of more than 250,000 deaths annually. Other estimates put that number above 400,000. According to the Agency for Health Care Research and Quality (AHRQ) 10% to 12% of patients experience an adverse event, and half of these are considered preventable.

Nurses play an integral role in patient safety and spend the most amount of time with patients. For example, according to a 2018 study, nurses account for 86% of all patient-facing time in ICUs, with only 13% of that time devoted to physicians.

Essential Facts

Critical thinking, clinical judgment, and reasoning are clearly related to patient outcomes, and improving these cognitive skills in nurses will decrease medical errors and improve patient safety and outcomes.

This chapter highlights the significance of patient safety and adverse outcomes. An overview of the initiatives implemented by TJC, the IOM, and QSEN are also included.

THE BIG PICTURE

Patient safety and quality of care are integral to all healthcare organizations and multiple agencies have developed comprehensive initiatives to improve patient outcomes and decrease the number of adverse events. However, in 1999, the IOM's *To Err Is Human: Building a Safer Health System* estimated the cost of medical errors was between $17 billion and $29 billion at hospitals across the country, with death rates between 44,000 and 98,000. This report highlighted the overall scope of the problem and various agencies, such as the IOM and TJC, created new initiatives to address these unacceptable rates of errors. However, a recent review by Daniel (2016) found that 250,000 deaths per year are due to medical errors, the third-highest cause of death in the United States, and that medical errors are underreported.

ADVERSE EVENTS

Adverse events have been described as an event that occurs because of medical care that could be considered preventable or nonpreventable. These include events that result in harm that is temporary or permanent (Harris, 2021), longer hospital stays, or death. Other events include "never events," such as wrong-side surgery, and "temporary events," such as an allergic reaction (U.S. Department of Health and Human Services/Office of the Inspector General, 2012). Adverse events take place in all healthcare settings; however, the Office of the Inspector General found that 21% of Medicare patients in long-term care hospitals experienced an adverse event, which is 46% higher than in hospitals, skilled nursing facilities, or rehabilitation hospitals (U.S. Department of Health and Human Services/Office of the Inspector General, 2018).

PATIENT SAFETY

According to the WHO (2020), patient safety is the absence of preventable harm and the reduction of the risk of unnecessary harm associated with healthcare to an acceptable minimum. An accepted minimum considers factors such as current knowledge and resources weighted against the risk of alternative treatments or nontreatment.

ASSESSING THE PROBLEM

Common Causes of Errors

In 2003, the AHRQ identified eight common causes of medical errors:

- Communication problems (verbal and written may occur at any juncture)
- Inadequate information flow (critical test results/coordination of medication transfer)
- Human problems (not following policies and procedures)
- Patient-related issues (improper ID, failure to obtain consent, inadequate patient education)
- Organizational transfer of knowledge (lack of training and orientation)
- Staffing patterns/workflow (inadequate staffing)
- Technical failures (equipment failure)
- Inadequate policies and procedures (lack of clearly written policies) (Always Culture, 2021)

FALLS

Patient falls continue to occur at alarming rates and often with devastating results. According to the AHRQ (2022) annual falls range from 750,000 to 1 million, with a rate of three to five falls per 1,000 bed days. Approximately one third of all in-patient hospital falls result in injury and include fractures and head injuries, which may be life-threatening. Weil (2015) examined falls from the 1950s to the present day and found that falls have increased during this period, which is related to an increase in patients who are older and have more comorbidities in addition to better reporting systems. Weil (2015) also posits that most safety committees have difficulty developing and implementing effective long-term aggressive fall prevention programs.

MEDICATION ERRORS

Medication errors may result in serious harm and are attributed to multiple factors and systematic breakdowns and occur in all settings. A medication error is defined as "any preventable event that may cause or lead to inappropriate medication use or patient harm while the medication is in the control of the healthcare professional, patient, or consumer," according to the National Coordinating Council for Medication Error Reporting and Prevention" (U.S. Food and Drug Administration, 2019, p. 1). According to Salar et al. (2020), medication errors are the sixth-leading cause of death in America. A recent meta-analysis revealed that 39% of errors were related to healthcare prescribers, 38% to nurses, and 23% to pharmacies. These statistics are alarming, and to date, the various policies and strategies that have been implemented have not mitigated the rates.

PRESSURE ULCERS

Pressure ulcers have been identified as one of the nursing quality indicators, and they fall under the auspices of nursing and have been correlated with poor nursing care (Ebi, 2020). Pressure ulcers are related to immobility, incontinence, and comorbidities and are correlated with infections, increased length of stay, and mortality. In the United States, 2.5 million people develop a pressure ulcer every year (AHRQ, 2020).

Essential Facts

Pressure ulcers are currently the most harmful and costly adverse events, with recent cost estimates of $26.8 billion per year. Furthermore, hospitals experience legal and financial burdens and costs associated with the prevention and treatment and a 1% reimbursement reduction from the Centers for Medicare and Medicaid for nosocomial pressure ulcers (Morse, 2019).

HOSPITAL-ACQUIRED INFECTIONS

Hospital-acquiredinfections (HAIs), or nosocomial infections, are infections that are usually acquired after hospitalization unless they were incubating prior to admission. They include Clostridium difficile infections (CDIs), hospital-acquired pneumonia (HAP), central line–associated bloodstream infections (CLABSIs), surgical site infections (SSIs), catheter-associated urinary tract infections (CAUTIs), and ventilator-associated pneumonia (VAP; Monegro et al., 2020). Although there are multiple mediating factors and nonadherence to infection control policies occurs across the healthcare setting and disciplines, Recio-Saucedo et al. (2018) completed a systematic review and found a direct correlation between missed nursing care and poor clinical outcomes.

Impact of COVID-19 on Patient Outcomes

In 2020, the unthinkable occurred with the emergence of COVID-19 and the pandemic that followed, which caused significant illness and death and changed our way of life in ways we could have never imagined. There was much uncertainty and fear and trial and error. Major interventions included quarantining, masks, and virtually shutting down society to flatten the curve. The development of vaccines and treatments changed the trajectory. Two years later, the number of cases has decreased, but we still live with uncertainty. Every facet of life has been impacted; however, the impact on healthcare and the resultant shortages across the various disciplines, especially nursing, have been significant. According to the AHRQ PSNet Annual Perspective (AHRQ, 2021) this novel virus disproportionately affected minorities, people with mental illness, the homeless, residents in long-term care facilities, the incarcerated, and people with comorbidities. The virus was so virulent that many people had to delay care and lifesaving treatments. In addition to workforce shortages, a lack of supplies, particularly personal protective equipment (PPE) complicated everything. A shift toward telehealth and workforce redesign was necessary to mitigate the spread. The effect on mental health across populations has been staggering in addition to the financial burdens we have all experienced. Some of the effects have not been quantified, and the long-term impacts are yet to be seen. According to Fleisher et al. (2022), there has been a severe decline in health care safety since the pandemic began. They further posit that the U.S. healthcare system is lacking and that there is a need to build a system that can maintain a culture of safety even in a pandemic. In support of this recent reports identify a correlation between the pandemic and infection control across healthcare settings, with increased percentages of infections in central lines (60%), CAUTI (44%), and increased incidence of methicillin-resistant *Staphylococcus aureus* (MRSA; 43%; Masson, 2022).

PATIENT SAFETY INITIATIVES

Adverse events and poor patient outcomes place myriad burdens on the healthcare system, with high morbidity and mortality rates among the most alarming. The financial burdens are staggering, despite multiple agencies implementing a wide array of strategies.

THE JOINT COMMISSION INITIATIVES

TJC is a global organization that focuses on patient safety and quality of care. Its mission is to improve healthcare and "inspire healthcare organizations to excel in providing safe and effective care of the highest quality and value" (TJC, 2022, para. 2). In 2003, TJC released the first patient safety goals. The original six goals were focused on the following:

- Patient identification
- Effective communication
- High-alert medications
- Eliminated wrong-side/site surgery
- Infusion pump safety
- Effectiveness of clinical alarms (JCAHO, 2003)

Every year TJC (2021a) continues to add new patient safety goals that healthcare facilities must address as part of their accreditation process. There are now 15 patient safety goals (see www.jointcommission.org/standards/national-patient-safety-goals/hospital-national-patient-safety-goals). They are also specific to the type of healthcare setting and now include infections, anticoagulant therapy, and a standardized protocol for preventing wrong-side/site surgery. Patient misidentification continues to be addressed and still occurs at unacceptable rates. According to TJC (2020), wrong-patient errors occur at all different stages of diagnosis and treatment. According to Choudhury and Vu (2020), it is challenging to detect; however, a review of a root-cause analysis by the Veteran's Administration found that out of 253 errors in the test cycle, 182 of them were related to patient misidentification. Furthermore, a survey of healthcare administrators found that 64% of them believe that the percentage of these types of errors are higher than the industry reported 8% to 10%. Clearly, there is still much work to do in achieving patient safety goals across all healthcare settings.

QUALITY AND SAFETY EDUCATION FOR NURSES

The QSEN competencies were created to address patient safety and improve patient outcomes. The Robert Wood Johnson Foundation funded the study, and a group of nursing experts collaborated to develop the QSEN competencies. There were four phases with specific criteria, and the website (https://qsen.org/) offers a plethora of strategies for helping students and nurses develop the knowledge, skills, and attitudes to incorporate the competencies in their practice settings. There are six competencies for the undergraduate and graduate nurse:

- Patient-centered care
- Teamwork and Collaboration
- Evidence-based Practice (EBP)
- Quality Improvement
- Safety
- Informatics (Hunt, 2012; QSEN, 2021)

NATIONAL ACADEMY OF MEDICINE

The National Academy of Medicine (NAM) was founded as the IOM in 1970. It is one of the three academies that make up the national academies. In partnership with the National Academy of Sciences, the National Academy of Engineering, and other stakeholders, the NAM draws on expertise across disciplines and domains to advance science, medicine, technology, and health. Its mission is to improve health, and its vision is a healthier future for all (NAM, 2021). In 1999, the IOM released its landmark report *To Err is Human: Building a Better Healthcare System,* in which it reported on the staggering fact that 98,000 died from preventable medical errors in the United States every year. In the past 20 years, initiatives have been implemented and progress has been made, but tens of thousands of patients are still being affected by preventable medical errors. The goal of achieving zero harm to patients is ambitious; however, improvements have been made in several areas (Association of American Medical Colleges, 2019; Table 1.1).

These interventions and results were significant; however, current outcomes need to be correlated with interventions to reach the goal "zero harm" to patients (TJC, 2022a). In support of this goal, Press Ganey (2020) has developed a new initiative Safety 2025: Accelerate to Zero, aimed at reducing patient and caregiver harm by 80% over the next five years.

The Institute for Healthcare Improvement focuses on quality improvement and outcomes. The institute

Table 1.1

Examples of Successful Initiatives

Agency	Initiative	Outcomes
AHRQ	National Scorecard on Hospital Acquired Conditions	2014–2017 20,000 lives saved
The Joint Commission	National Patient Safety Goals	Initiative in 2011 18-month effort to reduce falls across the country = 62% reduction in falls
Institute of Healthcare Improvement	Save 100,000 lives	Over 18 months there were 122,000 fewer deaths
World Health Organization (WHO)	Safe Surgery Save Lives Checklist (2009)	Participating hospitals' death rate reduced by 50%
Affordable Care Act (2010)	The Partnership of Patients (2010–2015)	"In 2016, the Department of Health and Human Services reported that the partnership and other government initiatives had contributed to 125,000 fewer patient deaths from hospital-acquired conditions between 2010 and 2015" (Haskins, 2019).

was created in 1991; its mission is to improve health and healthcare globally, and its vision is that everyone will have the best healthcare (IHI, 2021).

The PSQ Advisory (2021) was founded by Ann Scott Blouin to offer a strategic perspective on the relationship between excellence in quality and safety and financial security.

SUMMARY

Each year myriad patients experience an adverse event that may result in serious harm. Patient safety and quality of care continue to be addressed by all healthcare agencies with some promising outcomes. Progress has been made in some areas, but the rates are still alarmingly high, and we have a long way to go to reach "zero harm." This chapter highlighted the issues and provided a brief overview of the various initiatives undertaken to improve patient outcomes.

VIGNETTE

Terri Green is a new nurse who has just finished her formal orientation. She is very organized, but due to several the fact that several patients had complications, she started to rush and almost administered the wrong medication to the patient in the other bed. She quickly realized her mistake and administered the correct medications to the correct patient. Would this be considered an error? If so, what type of error? Should she report it?

Discussion Questions

1. Select one of the QSEN competencies and discuss how it can be applied in healthcare settings to decrease patient errors.

2. What is a root cause analysis? Why is it done?
3. Discuss the current initiatives and findings of TJC about patient safety.
4. Describe the nursing quality indicators and their significance.
5. Identify the most common nosocomial infections. What strategies have been employed at your healthcare organization to decrease these types of infections?

TIPS FROM THE FIELD

7 Tips for Improving Patient Safety:

- Focus on reducing readmissions (staffing ratios, discharge planning, transition to care)
- Reduce transmission of superbugs with hygiene and surveillance
- Improve transitions of care (www.jointcommission.org/standards)
- Reduce adverse drug events (follow safety protocols)
- Minimizing hospital-acquired infections (hand hygiene campaigns)
- Develop a policy for "never events" (apologize to family; conduct a root cause analysis)
- Compare policies to evidence-based guidelines

(www.healthcaredive.com/news/7-tips-for-improving-patient-safety-in-hospitals/421712)

SPECIAL TOPICS: SENTINEL EVENTS

What is a sentinel event? According to TJC (2022b) a sentinel event is one that results in death, permanent harm, or severe temporary harm. TJC works closely with hospitals to help prevent these types of occurrences.

The following are the most frequently reviewed sentinel events:

- Falls
- Unintended retention of a foreign object (URFO)
- Suicide
- Wrong surgery
- Delay in treatment

Additional sentinel events include

- unanticipated death of a full-term infant,
- discharge of an infant to the wrong family,
- abduction of any patient, and
- any patient elopement.

(www.jointcommission.org/resources/patient-safety-topics/sentinel-event/#:~:text=A%20sentinel%20event%20is%20a,harm%2C%20or%20severe%20temporary%20harm)

SUGGESTED CLASSROOM OR UNIT-BASED ASSIGNMENT

Interview a member of the quality improvement team at your healthcare organization. What is this member's specific role? What are the most common errors they see? What strategies do they believe are the most beneficial?

CASE EXEMPLAR 1.1: QSEN COMPETENCIES

Debra A. Simons, PhD, RN

In nursing education, evaluation is an important process used to measure student learning outcomes. Evaluation of students learning outcomes is an ongoing challenge for nurse educators. Nursing faculty are responsible for obtaining information for making value judgments about the quality of student learning and their competence in clinical practice. Collecting the right information about competencies in knowledge, skills, and attitudes is necessary for evaluation. The evaluation methods in clinical courses should provide data elements that provide information on how well students are meeting or have met the clinical objectives or competencies.

Nurse educators should incorporate QSEN competencies in their program outcomes and evaluation methods. The development of a clinical evaluation tool that incorporates the six QSEN competencies will assist nurse educators in gathering information on quality and safety when making value judgments about learners. A progression scale that includes expected behaviors allows student learners to make progress toward their learning as they progress through the program.

The Clinical Evaluation Tool

In addition to demographic data and course number and level, students are rated based on QSEN competencies on a proficiency scale of 0 to 4 (see Table 1.2). Based on the course level, points are converted (see Table 1.3). Examples of student expected behaviors are illustrated within each competency (see Table 1.4) and included in the evaluation tool.

Table 1.2

Proficiency Scale
How often does the student require the following:
1. Guidance
2. Direction
3. Monitoring
4. Support

(*continued*)

Table 1.2

Proficiency Scale (*continued*)

How often does the student exhibit the following:

1. A focus on the client or system
2. Accuracy, safety, and skillfulness
3. Assertiveness and initiative
4. Efficiency and organization
5. An eagerness to learn

SELF-DIRECTED: 4	
Almost never requires (less than 10% of the time)	Almost always exhibits (more than 90% of the time)
SUPERVISED: 3	
Occasionally requires (25% of the time) Very often exhibits (75% of the time)	
ASSISTED: 2	
Often requires (50% of the time)	Often exhibits (50% of the time)
NOVICE: 1	
Very often requires (75% of the time)	Occasionally exhibits (25% of the time)
DEPENDENT: 0	
Almost always requires (more than 90% of the time)	Very rarely exhibits (less than 10% of the time)

Table 1.3

Point Conversion Scale

Course	Pass	Need Improvement	Warning	Fail
Fundamental Nursing	2	1	0	0
Medical-Surgical Nursing	3	2	<2	0
Medical-Surgical II Nursing	3/4	<3	<2	0

Table 1.4

Example of Behaviors Demonstrating Competencies

Patient-Centered Care: Recognize the patient or designee as the source of control and full partner in providing compassionate and coordinated care based on respect for the patient's preferences, values, and needs.

- Identify opportunities for teaching health promotion, risk reduction, and disease prevention and incorporates patient education into the patient's plan of care.
- Practice therapeutic communication in developing a trusting nurse–patient relationship. Establishes professional boundaries in the care of patients
- Identify patient barriers to effective communication.
- Integrate holistic care and ethical principles that are sensitive and compassionate into the care of patients and families.
- Demonstrate sensitivity to cultural influences on the individual's reactions to the illness. Advocate for and empower the patient/family as partners in the care process and support their right to safe, compassionate, and holistic nursing care.

Teamwork and Collaboration: Function effectively within nursing and inter-professional teams, fostering open communication, mutual respect, and shared decision-making to achieve quality patient care.

- Demonstrate professional collaboration with members of the interdisciplinary healthcare team to improve patient outcomes.
- Utilize the EMR to foster interdisciplinary communication for consistency in patient care and patient safety.
- Participate in interprofessional rounding.
- Provide assistance to peers and the healthcare team to support teamwork and reduce or avoid errors.
- Delegate as appropriate to team members within their scope of practice.
- Model IMSAFE behaviors as outlined in TeamSTEPPS.
- Communicate professionally with patients/families, healthcare team, and peers.
- Participate in post-conferences and support peers in civil discourse.
- Applies TeamSTEPPS communication tools to clinical situations as appropriate.

(*continued*)

Table 1.4

Example of Behaviors Demonstrating Competencies (*continued*)

Evidence-Based Practice (EBP): Integrate best current evidence with clinical expertise and patient/family preferences and values for delivery of optimal health care.

- Integrate EBP in patient care delivery to support safe, quality patient care.
- Actively seek appropriate resources to answer clinical questions.
- Integrate best current evidence with clinical expertise, clinical data, and patient/family preferences and values for delivery of optimal health care.
- Apply essential patient/family information in the plan of care or teaching plan.
- Demonstrate knowledge of and adheres to evidence-based standards of care/policies/protocols for the institution.

Quality Improvement (QI): Use data to monitor the outcomes of care processes and use improvement methods to design and test changes to continuously improve the quality and safety of health care systems.

- Demonstrate awareness of and actively participates in the unit's quality improvement program.
- Identify practice gaps and opportunities for improvement within the clinical site/organization.
- Analyze the impact of factors such as access, cost, or team functioning on patient safety and quality improvement project efforts.

Safety: Minimize risk of harm to patients and providers through both system effectiveness and individual performance.

- Protect patient privacy and confidentiality in all communications (verbal, written, electronic).
- Use proper PPE and adhere to infection control procedures and policies. Demonstrate proper hand hygiene technique.
- Demonstrate competent use of medical devices in the care of a patient.
- Complete orientation to unit equipment.
- Use equipment per standards for safe patient assessment and monitoring.
- Identify personal gaps in knowledge and skill and seek help.

(*continued*)

Table 1.4

Example of Behaviors Demonstrating Competencies (*continued*)

- Use proper body mechanics and assistive devices to promote safe patient handling and avoid personal injury.
- Demonstrate safe medication administration.
- Use credible resources for researching medication information.
- Accurately record medication administration and monitor, report, and document the patient's response to the medication.
- Initially calculate correct dose and IV rate of administration prior to then using pump technology or other technology as a safety check.
- Identify IV compatibility and medication dilution.
- Describe the indication, action, and side effects of medications.
- Provide appropriate patient education on medications and medication safety to the patient/family.

Informatics: Use information and technology to communicate, manage knowledge, mitigate error, and support decision-making.

- Seek education about how information is managed in care settings before providing care.
- Apply technology and information management tools to support safe processes of care.
- Navigate the electronic health record.
- Document and plan patient care in an electronic health record.
- Employ communication technologies to coordinate care for patients.
- Use information management tools to monitor the outcomes of care processes.

Expected Outcomes: Allowing the student to participate in the evaluation process is important. Students should complete a self-assessment at the time of the formative and summative evaluation. Examples of expected behaviors should be included on the Clinical Evaluational Tool (CET) so students can see examples of the expected behaviors.

RESOURCES

Agency for Health Care Research and Quality (AHRQ). (2021). *AHRQ PSNet annual perspective: Impact of the COVID-19 pandemic on patient safety*. https://psnet.ahrq.gov/perspective/ahrq-psnet-annual-perspective-impact-covid-19-pandemic-patient-safety

AHC MEDIA. (2018). Joint Commission advisory addresses ensuring accurate patient identification. *Same-Day Surgery, 42*(12). https://www.ahrq.gov/patient-safety/resources/pstools/index.html

American Association of Critical-Care Nurses. (2021). *QSEN module learning series.* https://www.aacnnursing.org/Faculty/Teaching-Resources/QSEN/QSEN-Learning-Module-Series

Cappelleri, J. C., Zou, K. H., Bushmakin, A. G., Alvir, J. M. J., Alemayehu, D., & Symonds, T. (2014). *Patient-reported outcomes: Measurement, implementation, and interpretation.* CRC Press. https://doi.org/10.1201/b16139

Committee on Measuring the Impact of Interprofessional Education on Collaborative Practice and Patient Outcomes; Board on Global Health; Institute of Medicine. (2015). *Measuring the impact of interprofessional education on collaborative practice and patient outcomes.* National Academies Press. https://www.ncbi.nlm.nih.gov/books/NBK338360/ doi: 10.17226/21726 https://www.pso.ahrq.gov/

Disch, J., & Barnsteiner, J. (2021). QSEN in an Amazon World. *American Journal of Nursing, 121*(3), 40–46. https://doi.org/10.1097/01.NAJ.0000737176.16228.97.

Fleisher, L. A., Schreiber, M., Cardo, D., & Srinivasan, A. (2022). Health care safety during the pandemic and beyond—Building a system that ensures resilience. *New England Journal of Medicine, 386*(7), 609–611. http://dx.doi.org/10.1056/NEJMp2118285

Institute of Medicine. (2015). *Measuring the impact of interprofessional education on collaborative practice and patient outcomes.* The National Academies Press.

Masson, G. (2022). *Sharp drop in patient safety, infection control amid pandemic: 3 new findings.* https://www.beckershospitalreview.com/infection-control/sharp-drop-in-patient-safety-seen-amid-pandemic-3-findings.html

Patient Safety Movement. (2019). *The history of the patient safety movement.* https://psnet.ahrq.gov/primer/patient-safety-101

QSEN. (2021). Resources. https://qsen.org/faculty-resources/organizations/

Waterson, P. (2018). *Patient safety culture: Theory, methods and application.* CRC Press.

REFERENCES

Agency for Healthcare Quality and Research. (2020). *Pressure ulcers*. https://www.ahrq.gov/topics/pressure-ulcers.html

Agency for Healthcare Quality and Research. (2021). *AHRQ PSNet annual perspective: Impact of the COVID-19 pandemic on patient safety*. https://psnet.ahrq.gov/perspective/ahrq-psnet-annual-perspective-impact-covid-19-pandemic-patient-safety

Agency for Healthcare Quality and Research. (2022). *AHRQ's patient safety initiative: building foundations, reducing risk*. https://www.ahrq.gov/patients-co0nsumers/care-planning/errors/20tips/index.html

Always Culture. (2021). *The 8 most common root causes of medical errors*. https://alwaysculture.com/hcahps/communication-medications/8-most-common-causes-of-medical-errors/; https://archive.ahrq.gov/research/findings/final-reports/pscongrpt/psini2.html

Choudhury, L., & Vu, C. (2020). *Patient identification errors: A systems challenge*. Patient Safety Network AHRQ. https://psnet.ahrq.gov/web-mm/patient-identification-errors-systems-challenge. https://www.aamc.org/news-insights/20-years-patient-safety

Daniel, M. (2016). *Study suggests medical errors now third leading cause of death in the U.S.* https://www.hopkinsmedicine.org/news/media/releases/study_suggests_medical_errors_now_third_leading_cause_of_death_in_the_us?preview=true

Ebi, W. E., Hirko, G. F., & Mijena, D. A. (2019). Nurses' knowledge to pressure ulcer prevention in public hospitals in Wollega: A cross-sectional study design. *BMC Nursing, 18*, Article 20. https://doi.org/10.1186/s12912-019-0346-y

Haskins, J. (2018). *20 years of patient safety*. AAMC. https://www.aamc.org/news-insights/20-years-patient-safety

Hunt, D. (2012). RN QSEN competencies: A bridge to practice. *Nursing Made Incredibly Easy!, 10*(5), 1–3. https://doi.org/10.1097/01.NME.0000418040.92006.70

Institute of Healthcare Initiatives. (2021). *About us*. http://www.ihi.org/about/Pages/innovationscontributions.aspx

Institute of Medicine. (1999). *To err is human: Building a safer health system*. Washington, DC: National Academies Press.

Joint Commission on Accreditation of Healthcare Organizations. (2003). JCAHO national patient safety goals. *Kans Nurse, 78*(6), 7–8.

Morse, S. (2019). Pressure ulcers cost the health system $26.8 billion a year. *Healthcare Finance*. https://www.healthcarefinancenews.com/news/pressure-ulcers-cost-health-system-268-billion-year

National Academy of Medicine. (2021). *About us*. https://nam.edu/about-the-nam/

Press Ganey. (2020). *Press Ganey launches groundbreaking safety initiative to advance the industry toward zero harm*. https://www.pressganey.com/about/news/press-ganey-launches-groundbreaking-safety-initiative-to-advance-the-industry-toward-zero-harm

Quality and Safety Education for Nurses (QSEN). (2021). https://qsen.org/about-qsen/qsen-history/

Recio-Saucedo, A., Dall'Ora, C., Maruotti, A., Ball, J., Briggs, J., Meredith, P., Redfern, O. C., Kovacs, C., Prytherch, D., Smith, G. B., & Griffiths, P. (2018). What impact does nursing care left undone have on patient outcomes? Review of the literature. *Journal of Clinical Nursing, 27*(11–12), 2248–2259. https://doi.org/10.1111/jocn.14058

Salar, A., Kiani, F., & Rezaee, N. (2020). Preventing the medication errors in hospitals: A qualitative study. *International Journal of Africa Nursing Sciences*. https://www.sciencedirect.com/science/article/pii/S2214139120301128#:~:text=A%20recent%20meta%2Danalysis%20study,Al%2DWorafi%2C%202020

Stocking, J. C., Sandrock, C., Fitall, E., Hall, K. K., & Gale, B. (n.d.).

The Joint Commission. (2020). *National Patient Safety Goals effective July 2020 for the hospital program*. https://www.ncsbn.org/Facts_about_National_Patient_Safety_Goals.pdf

The Joint Commission. (2021a). *National patient safety goals*. https://www.jointcommission.org/standards/national-patient-safety-goals/hospital-national-patient-safety-goals/

The Joint Commission. (2021b). *About the joint commission.* https://www.jointcommission.org/about-us/

The Joint Commission. (2022a). *Leading the way to zero.* https://www.jointcommission.org/performance-improvement/joint-commission/leading-the-way-to-zero/

The Joint Commission. (2022b). *Sentinel event.* https://www.jointcommission.org/resources/patient-safety-topics/sentinel-event/#:~:text=A20sentinel20event20is20a,providers20involved20in20the20event.

U.S. Department of Health and Human Services/Office of the Inspector General. (2012). *Spotlight on adverse events.* https://oig.hhs.gov/reports-and-publications/archives/spotlight/2012/adverse.asp

U.S. Department of Health and Human Services/Office of the Inspector General. (2018). *Adverse events in long-term-care hospitals: National incidence among Medicare beneficiaries.* https://oig.hhs.gov/oei/reports/oei-06-14-00530.asp

U.S. Food and Drug Administration. (2019). *Working to reduce medication errors.* https://www.fda.gov/drugs/information-consumers-and-patients-drugs/working-reduce-medication-errors

Weil, T. P. (2015). Patient falls in hospitals: An increasing problem. *Geriatric Nursing, 36*(5), 342–347. https://doi-org.rdas-proxy.mercy.edu/10.1016/j.gerinurse.2015.07.004

World Health Organization. (2019). *WHO calls for urgent action to reduce patient harm in healthcare.* https://www.who.int/news-room/detail/13-09-2019-who-calls-for-urgent-action-to-reduce-patient-harm-in-healthcare

World Health Organization. (2020). *Patient safety.* https://www.who.int/patientsafety/en/

2

Primary Causes of Adverse Events in Nursing

You don't need to know the whole alphabet of Safety. The a, b, c of it will save you if you follow it: Always Be Careful.

—Colorado School of Mines Magazine

There are many causes of adverse events across healthcare institutions, and several are highly correlated with nursing care. Medication administration errors continue to persist despite the various strategies employed by healthcare institutions and agencies. These include poor communication, medication administration errors, misuse of technology, poorly conceived processes and execution, and workload issues.

In this chapter, you will learn:

1. The relationship between poor communication
2. Types of medication administration errors
3. Issues with misuse of technology
4. Poorly conceived processes and execution
5. How workload issues correlate with adverse events

POOR COMMUNICATION

One of the major causes of adverse events is related to issues with communication. These types of errors that occur across healthcare institutions cost approximately $1.7 billion per year and are related to miscommunication, not recording information, ignoring messages, or never receiving them. The three most prevalent communication breakdowns are poor documentation, miscommunication about a patient's condition, and failure to read the medical record (White, 2016). A report by CRICO Strategies (2015) on medical malpractice claims analyzed 674 nursing cases. For the 2015 report, CRICO analyzed more than 23,000 medical malpractice claims and lawsuits filed between 2009 and 2013 in which a patient experienced some degree of harm. Nurses were named in 647 of the cases analyzed. CRICO found that 75% of the communication errors occurred in an inpatient setting, and the most frequently cited factors were failure to patient conditions, unsympathetic response to patient complaints, and poor documentation of clinical findings (Beckers, 2016). A cross-sectional study done in Turkey found that 23% of the sample approximately 50% of the physicians and nurses had experienced a medical error due to an issue with communication (Topcu et al., 2017). Galatzan and Harrington (2018) posit that 80% of adverse events in healthcare are related to miscommunication. Poor communication and a lack of teamwork and collaboration were attributed to 72% of adverse events in maternity care (Rönnerhag et al., 2019). However, Clapper and Chinn (2020) conducted a systematic review and concluded that most errors were attributed to errors of omission or commission, not miscommunication. This is in opposition to what others have found but does merit further exploration.

Although the data may offer some conflicting results, effective communication is vital. A particular area for communication errors is during patient hand-off or change of shift. Bakon et al. (2017) identify this time as a time as one that is widely recognized for potential patient errors as important information may not be communicated.

Essential Facts

In 2006, The Joint Commission (TJC) established a national patient safety goal to address patient hand-offs and in 2010 it became a standard (TJC, 2017).

MEDICATION ADMINISTRATION

Medication errors continue to be a serious concern and are related to many different factors. Medication administration is one of the most frequently performed tasks of nurses and is a frequent cause of adverse events (Cottell et al., 2020). According to Abdalla et al. (2020), medication administration errors are a global problem and may result in an increase in morbidity and mortality and cause financial burdens (Slawomirski et al., 2017). Some of the main causes of nurse related medication errors include failure to properly identify the patient, heavy workloads, staff shortages, noise and distractions, fatigue, sound-alike drugs, the misuse of abbreviations, an illegible prescriptions, inappropriate dosage and infusion rates, incorrect time, and poor communication during change of shift. Worldwide, medication errors are one of the most common errors and are frequently not reported. A review of medication errors was analyzed by Björkstén et al. (2016) nursing malpractice cases in Sweden and found that they were related most often to "wrong dose" followed by "wrong drug," "wrong patient," and "omission." Individual contributing factors included negligence, not following protocol, practice beyond scope, and inappropriate communication. Systemic factors included role overload, look-alike meds, unclear orders, and interruptions. Nurses with less than 2 years of experience were more likely to make an error due to a lack of knowledge, with the wrong patient and the wrong drug administered being most common. The authors posit that this is like other countries. To address these issues, workplaces must have patient safety processes and continuing education (Björkstén et al., 2016). According to Svitlica et al. (2017), medication errors are the most common preventable adverse event that occurs in the hospital. Factors that contribute to medication errors can be divided into failures by health professionals, which include a host of errors that often relate to not following the long-established "rights of medication administration"; a lack of knowledge, skills, and attitudes about safe medication administration; or system failures or missions. Failures within the system include poor communication, inadequate staffing, vague authorization, more complex technologies, and a focus on reducing expenses.

Berdot et al. (2016) identify prescription, delivery, and administration as the three main areas where a medication error can occur. Nurses are the last line of defense in medication administration, and despite various interventions, errors continue to persist. Medication errors occur worldwide. A discussion of medication errors in Ireland highlights those errors are multidisciplinary and can be made by the prescriber, pharmacists, nurses, and patients and can happen at any point in the medication management process. There is a system of checks and balances whereby the order is prescribed, then verified and dispensed by the pharmacist, and then reviewed and verified again by the nurse. However, errors abound with incorrect orders, dosages, drug selection, omissions, neglecting to check for allergies and other areas of the patient's history, and wrong routes and times (Leufer & Joanne, 2013). According to Hung et al. (2015), in Taiwan, administering wrong oral medication occurs twice as often as patient falls and posited that scholars have identified the structure of the nursing unit and nursing errors; however, few studies have been done in this area. Wright (2010) completed a review of the literature to explore the relationship between miscalculation and medication errors and concluded there was insufficient evidence in this area. Errors by nursing students and near-miss errors are another area of concern, and according to Kennedy (2017) they are underreported, and many schools do not have a clear process for addressing and tracking errors by nursing students. These data span the past 10 years and highlight that many of these issues persist. In the following chapters, additional strategies for preventing medication errors are highlighted.

MISUSE OF TECHNOLOGY AND ADVERSE OUTCOMES

The continued development of technology and technological advances has had a significant impact on healthcare across the disciplines. While it has improved patient safety it has also had negative unforeseen consequences (Singh & Sittig, 2016; Nielsen & Barratt, 2009). Throughout the years, healthcare institutions (Quinn, 2016) have incorporated cutting-edge technology as it has become available. Health information technology (Health IT) has certainly changed the way healthcare is delivered and, in many ways, has improved patient outcomes, but it has also been correlated with negative patient outcomes. Major areas of concern related to hardware or software that malfunctions. For example, the electronic health record (EHR) system could be breached or have a glitch. There always needs to be a backup system in case this occurs. Another issue is the misuse of technology due to human error. Healthcare providers may not fully understand how to use the technology, or they may ignore warnings or alarms. Alarm fatigue has been well documented; for example, the IV pump alarms go off frequently, and it becomes part of the background noise and does not get the attention it needs. Another area is the lack of oversight and identification of potential risks. Due to the high rate of errors in medication administration, there has been a variety of technology, such as the Pyxis system, electronic medication administration, and barcoding. However, there can be errors with all these systems. The pharmacist might place the wrong medication or dose in the Pyxis bin, and if the nurse who is administering it does not read it three times, they might not administer the wrong medication. The barcoding might not be used, and incorrect medication might be administered to the wrong patient (Singh & Siggit, 2016). It is important to remember that technology is a tool and does not replace oversight by the various healthcare providers. Kim et al. (2017) conducted a systematic review on problems with Health IT and patient outcomes. They examined 34 qualitative studies and identified similar issues that have been previously associated with safety and Health It. They identified poor user interface led to miscommunication and errors of commission. They also identified that issues with delayed care, system access, system updates, and system functionality were related to clinical errors. They found a correlation between IT problems and patient harm and death. And in 10 out of the 34 studies, near-miss events were reported. Because mainly qualitative studies were included in their analysis, they recommend further quantitative research to identify more specific correlations.

A jarring example of misuse of technology and the significance of healthcare providers having the knowledge and critical thinking and logic is an incident where a 16-year-old boy was prescribed Septra, which is a once-per-day dose, but the EHR incorrectly listed it as 38.5. The physician, pharmacist, and nurse carried out the order exactly as it was recommended in the EHR, which resulted in the patient receiving 38.5 doses at one time and was administered one pill at a time. The error was discovered when the patient complained of tingling, confusion, and feeling numb all over. How does an error like this happen? Technology is still fraught with issues with unfriendly user interfaces, alert fatigue, and the ability to use cut and paste features when documenting information in the electronic medical record (Vélez-Díaz-Pallarés et al., 2017).

POORLY CONCEIVED PROCESSES AND EXECUTION

Every procedure requires a process with specific guidelines or steps one should take when carrying out or executing an order. If the process is not clearly stated or the steps in the process are not followed, an error may occur. A common root cause of a medical error is related to poorly written or inadequate policies, which can lead to a disruption in processes and execution of procedures (Dufilho, 2017). Medication errors may be identified as errors in executing the plan or planning errors (Wittich et al., 2014). Safeguarding processes can decrease patient errors. Patient errors can occur throughout the process. When an error occurs, the process, rather than the person, is analyzed to determine the root cause (World Health Organization, 2019). Many systematic errors can be prevented with better policies and practice (Slawomirski et al., 2017). Policies and procedures should be developed based on current evidence, and the healthcare team must receive ongoing training and education with continual oversight.

WORKLOAD ISSUES

Workload issues in nursing and healthcare have been the subject of much discussion and debate (Schroers et al., 2021). While it is well known that there is a strong relationship between staffing ratios and staffing mix and patient outcomes, there is less certainty regarding the optimal staffing ratios (Brennan et al., 2013); however, there is a direct correlation between staffing levels and patient outcomes (Brennan et al., 2013; Duffield et al. 2011). Nurse–patient ratios have been the subject of much debate as to the optimal ratio. However, current evidence demonstrates a correlation between nurse–patient ratios and patient outcomes. "A great number of studies have been conducted to examine the relationship between nurse staffing and patient outcomes. It has been shown that lower nurse-to-patient ratio (better nurse staffing) and RN skill mix are related to better quality of patient care" (Aiken et al., 2011; Kalisch et al., 2012; Staggs et al., 2012, as cited in Shin et al., 2018). In their meta-analysis, Shin et al. (2018) concluded that adverse patient events were directly associated with patient-to-nurse ratios. Kane et al. (2007) found a relationship between RN staffing and lower mortality rates. When there were higher patient-to-staff ratios there is an increase in adverse events, such as hospital-acquired pneumonia. According to Cho et al. (2017), there is an improvement in patient outcomes, an increase in patient satisfaction, and a decrease in adverse events when there are adequate staffing ratios. Cho et al. (2017) conducted a study on staffing ratios, perception of missed care, and patient experiences. The average patient-to-nurse ratio was 11.5 patients per registered nurse. Nurse perceptions and patient perceptions varied regarding whether they believed this ratio was adequate; 77.4% of patients felt that there was adequate nursing staff, but only 10.2% of the nurses surveyed felt that staffing enabled them to provide quality care. The patients had higher scores than the nurses. However, they found that lower perceived staffing adequacy was associated with missed communication and lower ratings on care received. They were also correlated with adverse events and missed care. Because the data have been inconsistent and nurse-to-patient ratios vary, Rochefort et al. (2021) are conducting a longitudinal study that should be completed in 2024 and builds upon previous studies. "The objectives of this study are to (a) examine the associations between nurse staffing practices and the risk of adverse events (AEs); and (b) determine thresholds for safe nurse staffing" (Roth et al., 2017, p. 1567). This study has the potential to yield important results that can be used to determine optimal staffing and skill mix. Griffiths et al. (2018) completed a systematic review on staffing levels and adverse events. They posit that low nurse staffing levels are correlated with multiple adverse events and, most notably, mortality rates. However, despite the mounting evidence of adequate staffing ratios and patient outcomes, the causal link remains the subject of debate. The focus of their systematic review was on missed patient care, which has been identified as a beneficial way to evaluate if nurse-to-patient ratios are adequate. They found that low staffing is associated with missed nursing care in hospitals and although this requires further investigation could be a "promising indicator of nurse staffing adequacy" (Roth et al., 2017, p. 1474). Although there are other factors related to poor patient outcomes, workload and staffing are highly correlated with adverse events and it is vital to address this issue in all healthcare organizations.

SUMMARY

Common causes of adverse events addressed in this chapter include poor communication. Most of the literature reviewed demonstrated a relationship. Types and causes of medication errors were discussed. Types of errors include wrong medication, dose, route of administration, and misidentification of patients. Medication errors in addition to other errors have significant correlations with misuse of technology and poorly conceived processes and execution. The relationship between staffing levels and adverse events has been well established; however, this is still the subject of dispute and requires additional explorations.

VIGNETTE

The nurses on a medical-surgical unit are concerned about the high patient-to-staff ratios, which vary from 7 to 10 patients per day. What steps can the nurses take to advocate for adequate nurse-to-patient ratios? What data will they need? Which stakeholders do they need to contact?

Discussion Questions

1. Discuss common issues with miscommunication. What can be done to improve communication among healthcare workers?
2. Discuss the major causes of medication errors.
3. Discuss the positive and negative issues related to technology.
4. What are some ways that processes, execution procedures, and protocols can be improved?
5. What is the relationship between staffing ratios and patient outcomes and patient satisfaction?

TIPS FROM THE FIELD

Strategies for improving communication among healthcare workers:

- SBAR (Situation, Background, Assessment, Recommendation) Communication
- The STICC (Situation, Task, Intention, Concern, Calibrate) Protocol

Strategies for improving communication in healthcare conversations with patients:

- The Bathe (Background, Affect, Troubles, Handline, Empathetic Statement) Protocol
- The AWARE (Announce, Welcome, Ask, Review, Exit) Approach to Patient Interactions
- Patient Teach Back
- Patient Satisfaction
- New Communication Tools (smartphones, text messaging)

Visit www.hipaajournal.com/communication-strategies-in-healthcare for additional information on these protocols.

SPECIAL TOPICS: FOCUS ON MEDICATION SAFETY

10 Strategies to Reduce Medication Errors:

- Minimize clutter.
- Verify orders.
- Use barcodes.
- Be aware of sound-alike, look-alike drugs.
- Have a second pair of eyes check the orders.
- Involve the patient.
- Trust your gut.
- Be proactive.
- Design effective warning.
- Track medication orders.

(From "10 Strategies to Reduce Medication Errors," *Drug Topics Journal*, by Tzipora Lider, RPh, April 2020, *164(4)*, www.drugtopics.com/view/10-strategies-reduce-medication-errors.)

SUGGESTED CLASSROOM OR UNIT-BASED ASSIGNMENT

Develop a poster presentation on miscommunication and strategies to improve communication among healthcare workers.

CASE EXEMPLAR 2.1: TRANSPLANTS AND MISIDENTIFICATION

Scott Murphy

Case Presentation

In 2003, a transplant patient died due to receiving an incompatible ABO heart/lung transplant at Duke University Hospital. A root cause analysis was conducted and completed and identified as human error. The practitioners failed to correctly identify the ABO as being incompatible. The donor had a type A blood group, and the 17-year-old recipient had an O blood group. Shortly after transplant and removal from bypass, her organ function quickly deteriorated, and that is when they identified the error when the transplant immunology lab called to advise of the incompatibility in the blood group. She was stabilized and returned to the pediatric ICU, and three days later underwent a second transplant with the correct ABO. Despite all possible interventions, she incurred significant brain swelling from the initial insult and died (Fulkerson, 2003; Hopkins Tanne, 2003).

Analysis

The root cause analysis identified that the error was related to human error occurring at several points due to a lack of redundancy and inadequate policy and procedures that were in effect during that time.

The critical failure was the lack of a positive confirmation of ABO compatibility of the donor organs and the identified recipient patient (Fulkerson, 2003).

Corrective Action

Due to this event and previous misidentification in ABO compatibility, the policy and procedures were updated to prevent this type of error. The following procedure was developed by UNOS/OPTN (United Network for Organ Sharing/Organ Procurement and Transplant Network). There are identified as Policy 3.1.2).

The requirements are as follows:

- Upon receipt of an organ prior to implantation the transplant center is responsible for verifying the recorded donor ABO with the recorded ABO of the intended recipient (effective 2/1/04) and the UNOS Donor ID number (effective 9/1/07).
- The verification process has been modified and now requires multiple checks during the pre-recovery period the transplant surgeon along with a healthcare professional must separately identify the ABO and subtype of the donor.
- The recipient transplant process also must follow similar guidelines prior to transplant.

Summary

This patient exemplar highlights the need for adequate checks and balances in the healthcare setting to ensure patient safety. High-risk procedures require the healthcare team to be particularly diligent. It's always important to follow the policies and procedures that have been created due to instances like this. Evaluation and reinforcement of the policies and procedures should be done on an ongoing basis.

References

Fulkerson, W. (2003). *Duke releases letter to UNOS concerning Jesica Santillan. Duke Health News*, Duke University Hospital https://today.duke.edu/2003/02/fulkerson0203.html.

Hopkins, T. J. (2003). When Jesica died. *British Medical Journal, 326*(7391), 717.

CASE EXEMPLAR 2.2: A NURSE'S FIRST ADVERSE EVENT

Courtney Wallace, MSN, RN, CPHQ

Every nurse remembers their first adverse event. I remember every detail of mine even though it was over a decade ago. I was working the night shift on a cardiac stepdown unit and admitted an older woman at two in the morning. She insisted on taking her amitriptyline to help her sleep. Her daughter and I reviewed her medication list, and I faxed it to the pharmacy; this was before electronic medical records, and barcode medication scanning were widely used in rural areas. I pulled out the medication from Pyxis, and it prompted me to dispense six tablets for a total dose of 600 mg. This seemed excessive. I reviewed the medication book, called the pharmacist, and even double-checked with the family. Still feeling uncomfortable, I called the pharmacist again and verified with the provider. By this time, the pharmacist was irritated with my second call; the provider said, "Just give the medication and we can figure it out in the morning," and the patient was getting frustrated with the delay. Despite the uneasy feeling in the pit of my stomach, I had been reassured by multiple people, so, I gave the medication.

Two weeks later, I received an invite to attend a root cause analysis to determine the causes of an overdose of amitriptyline for the patient I admitted. For 5 nights following admission, a nurse gave six tablets of amitriptyline at bedtime. The patient had become more and more somnolent, and by the end of the week, she was unable to maintain her oxygen saturation and was intubated.

Once she was in the ICU, the amitriptyline was quickly thought to be the cause of her somnolence, and the medication was stopped. She slowly recovered and was ultimately discharged home with minimal lasting effects. At the root cause analysis, several potential causes were identified that led to that first dose and the continued administration of the medication. These included transcription error, dispensing error, a poorly defined and followed medication reconciliation process, a manual pharmacy process for verifying high dose medications, and poor communication and critical thinking regarding the patient's ongoing concern of mental status changes prior to the need for intubation.

Would this event have occurred today? I hope not. There are formal requirements for medication reconciliation, tighter control of high dose medications, and tools for clear communication, including SBAR. These are just some examples of processes and tools that aim to prevent adverse events; however, they are no substitute for the uneasy feeling in your gut. I implore you to learn from my mistake, listen to your gut, and speak up for safety.

RESOURCES

https://www.aacnnursing.org/AACN-Essentials

https://www.ismp.org/

https://www.ahrq.gov/patient-safety/resources/index.html

Mirjalili, N. (2020). Ethical leadership, nursing error and error reporting from the nurses' perspective. *Nursing Ethics*, *27*(2), 609–620. https://doi.org/10.1177/0969733019858706

Newman-Toker, D. E., McDonald, K. M., & Meltzer, D. O. (2013). How much diagnostic safety can we afford, and how should we decide? A health economics perspective. *BMJ Quality & Safety*, *22*(Suppl. 2), ii11–ii20.

REFERENCES

Abdalla, E., Abdoon, I., Osman, B., & Mohamed, E. (2020). Perception of medication errors' causes and reporting among Sudanese nurses in teaching hospitals. *Applied Nursing Research*, *51*, 151207.

Bakon, S., Wirihana, L., Christensen, M., & Craft, J. (2017). Nursing handovers: An integrative review of the different models and processes available. *International Journal of Nursing Practice*, *23*(2). https://doi-org.rdas-proxy.mercy.edu/10.1111/ijn.12520 DOI: 10.1111/ijn.12520

Beckers. (2016). *5 things to know about communication errors, nurses and patient safety.* https://www.beckershospitalreview.com/quality/5-thing-to-know-about-communication-errors-nurses-and-patient-safety.html

Berdot, S., Roudot, M., Schramm, C., Katsahian, S., Durieux, P., & Sabatier, B. (2016). Interventions to reduce nurses' medication administration errors in inpatient settings: A systematic review and meta-analysis. *International Journal of Nursing Studies*, *53*, 342–350. https://doi.org/10.1016/j.ijnurstu.2015.08.012

Björkstén, K., Bergqvist, M., Andersén-Karlsson, E., Benson, L., & Ulfvarson, J. (2016). Medication errors as malpractice – A qualitative content analysis of 585 medication errors by nurses in Sweden. *BMC Health Services Research*, *16*(1), 431. https://doi.org/10.1186/s12913-016-1695-9

Brennan, C. W., Daly, B. J., & Jones, K. R. (2013). State of the science: The relationship between nurse staffing and patient outcomes. *Western Journal of Nursing Research*, *35*(6), 760–794.

Cho, S. H., Mark, B., Knafl, G., Hyoung, E. C., & Yoon, H. J. (2017). Relationships between nurse staffing and patients' experiences, and the mediating effects of missed nursing care. *Journal of Nursing Scholarship*, *49*(3), 347–355.

Clapper, T. C., & Ching, K. (2020). Debunking the myth that many medical errors are attributed to communication. *Medical Education*, *54*(1), 74–81. https://doi.org/10.1111/medu.13821

Cottell, M., Wätterbjörk, I., & Hälleberg Nyman, M. (2020). Medication-related incidents at 19 hospitals: A retrospective register study using incident reports. *Nursing Open*, *7*, 1526–1535. https://doi.org/10.1002/nop2.534 Funding information: https://www.oecd.org/health/health-systems/The-economics-of-patient-safety-March-2017.pdf

CRICO. (2015). *Malpractice Risks in Communication Failures.* https://www.rmf.harvard.edu/Malpractice-Data/Annual-Benchmark-Reports/Risks-in-Communication-Failures

Duffield, C., Diers, D., O'Brien-Pallas, L., Aisbett, C., Roche, M., King, M., & Aisbett, K. (2011). Nursing staffing, nursing workload, the work environment and patient outcomes. *Applied Nursing Research*, *24*(4), 244–255.

Dufilho, M. (2017). Give scripting a chance in medication administration. *Always Culture*. https://alwaysculture.com/page/2/?cat=-1

Galatzan, B. J., & Carrington, J. M. (2018). Exploring the state of the science of the nursing hand-off communication. *Computers, Informatics, Nursing*, *36*(10), 484–493. https://doi.org/10.1097/CIN.0000000000000461

Griffiths, P., Recio-Saucedo, A., Dall'Ora, C., Briggs, J., Maruotti, A., Meredith, P., Smith, G., & Ball, J. (2018). The association between nurse staffing and omissions in nursing care: A systematic review. *Journal of Advanced Nursing*, *74*(7), 1474–1487. https://doi.org/10.1111/jan.13564

Hung, C. C., Lee, B.-O., Tsai, S.-L., Tseng, Y. S., & Chang, C.-H. (2015). Structure determines medication errors in nursing units: A mechanistic approach. *West J Nurs Res, 37*(3), 299–319. doi: 10.1177/0193945913513849

Kane, R. L., Shamliyan, T. A., Mueller, C., Duval, S., & Wilt, T. J. (2007). The association of registered nurse staffing levels and patient outcomes: Systematic review and meta-analysis. *Medical Care, 45*(12), 1195–1204. http://dx.doi.org.libproxy.adelphi.edu/10.1097/MLR.0b013e3181468ca3

Kennedy, M. S. (2017). Tracking errors, assessing patients, redesigning processes—It's all about safe care. *American Journal of Nursing, 117*(10), 7. https://doi.org/10.1097/01.NAJ.0000525852.44945.ab

Kim, M. O., Coiera, E., & Magrabi, F. (2017). Problems with health information technology and their effects on care delivery and patient outcomes: A systematic review. *Journal of the American Medical Informatics Association, 24*(2), 246–250. https://doi.org/10.1093/jamia/ocw154

Leufer, T., & Joanne, C.-H. (2013). Let's do no harm: Medication errors in nursing: Part 1. *Nurse Education in Practice, 13*(3), 213–216.

Nielsen, S., & Barratt, M. J. (2009). Prescription drug misuse: Is technology friend or foe? *Drug and Alcohol Review, 28*, 81–86. https://doi.org/10.1111/j.1465-3362.2008.00004.x

Pérez, M. M., Dafonte, C., Pérez Boado, A. B., & Gómez, A. (2019). Tracking and minimization of adverse events in the patient care process while in a hospital emergency service area. *Proceedings, 31*(1), 48.

Quinn, R. (2016). Potential dangers of using technology in healthcare. *The Hospitalist.* https://www.the-hospitalist.org/hospitalist/article/121825/potential-dangers-using-technology-healthcare

Rochefort, C., Abrahamowicz, M., Biron, A., Bourgault, P., Gaboury, I., Haggerty, J., & McCusker, J. (2021). Nurse staffing practices and adverse events in acute care hospitals: The research protocol of a multisite patient-level longitudinal study. *Journal of Advanced Nursing, 77*(3), 1567–1577. https://doi.org/10.1111/jan.14710

Rönnerhag, M., Severinsson, E., Haruna, M., & Berggren, I. (2019). A qualitative evaluation of healthcare professionals' perceptions of adverse events focusing on communication and teamwork in maternity care. *Journal of Advanced Nursing, 75*(3), 585–593. https://doi.org/10.1111/jan.13864

Roth, C., Brewer, M., & Wieck, K. L. (2017). Using a Delphi method to identify human factors contributing to nursing errors. *Nursing Forum, 52*(3), 173–179. https://doi-org.rdas-proxy.mercy.edu/10.1111/nuf.12178

Schroers, G., Ross, J. G., & Moriarty, H. (2021). Nurses' perceived causes of medication administration errors: A qualitative systematic review. *Joint Commission Journal on Quality & Patient Safety, 47*(1), 38–53. https://doi-org.rdas-proxy.mercy.edu/10.1016/j.jcjq.2020.09.010

Shin, S., Park, J.-H., & Bae, S.-H. (2018). Nurse staffing and nurse outcomes: A systematic review and meta-analysis. *Nursing Outlook, 66*(3), 273–282.

Singh, H., & Sittig, D. F. (2016). Measuring and improving patient safety through health information technology: The Health IT Safety Framework. *BMJ Qual Saf, 25*(4), 226–32. doi: 10.1136/bmjqs-2015-004486

Slawomirski, L., Auraaen, A., & Klazinga, N. (2017). The economics of patient safety: Strengthening a value-based approach to reducing patient harm at national level. *OECD Health Working Papers*, (96). https://doi.org/10.1787/5a9858cd-en

Svitlica, B. B., Simin, D., & Milutinović, D. (2017). Potential causes of medication errors: Perceptions of Serbian nurses. *International Nursing Review, 64*(3), 421–427.

The Joint Commission. (2017). *Inadequate hand-off communication.* https://www.jointcommission.org/-/media/tjc/documents/resources/patient-safety-topics/sentinel-event/sea_58_hand_off_comms_9_6_17_final_(1).pdf?db=web&hash=5642D63C1A5017BD214701514DA00139

Topcu, I., Turkmen, A. S., Sahiner, N. C., Savaser, S., & Sen, H. (2017). Physicians' and nurses' medical errors associated with communication failures. *Journal of Pakistan Medical Association, 67*(4), 600–604.

Vélez-Díaz-Pallarés, M., Álvarez Díaz, A. M., Gramage Caro, T., Vicente Oliveros, N., Delgado-Silveira, E., Muñoz García, M., Cruz-Jentoft, A. J., & Bermejo-Vicedo, T. (2017). Technology-induced errors associated with computerized provider order entry software for older patients. *Int J Clin Pharm, 39*(4), 729–742. doi: 10.1007/s11096-017-0474-y

White, J. (2016). *How communication problems put patients, hospitals in jeopardy.* https://www.healthcarebusinesstech.com/communication-patient-harm/

Wittich, C. M., Burkle, C. M., & Lanier, W. L. (2014). Medication errors: An overview for clinicians. *Mayo Clin Proc, 89*(8), 1116–1125. doi: 10.1016/j.mayocp.2014.05.007

World Health Orgnization. (2019). *Patient safety.* Key Facts. https://www.who.int/news-room/fact-sheets/detail/patient-safety

Wright, K. (2010). Do calculation errors by nurses cause medication errors in clinical practice? A literature review. *Nurse Education Today, 30*(1), 85–97.

II

Improving Patient Safety and Decreasing Adverse Events

3

The Safe Practitioner

An incident is just the tip of the iceberg, a sign of a much larger problem below the surface.

– Don Brown

There are many potential causes of adverse events and poor outcomes; however, the practitioner plays a pivotal role in creating a culture of safety. The healthcare practitioner must have the knowledge, skills, and attitude to become a safe practitioner. This chapter focuses on the educational and developmental processes required to prepare nurses and other healthcare providers for providing complex care across the life span.

In this chapter, you will learn:

1. Ways to be a safe practitioner
2. Education and knowledge level and their relation to patient safety
3. Key components of the orientation process
4. Core competencies relating to safe practitioners
5. Importance of lifelong learning

ATTRIBUTES OF A SAFE PRACTITIONER

Patient outcomes are important to every single person in the healthcare system, and every individual and department must do their part and follow the process to promote positive patient outcomes. The focus of this book is on nursing, and the role of nurses in this system is highlighted. Nurses are central to the healthcare team as they spend more time with patients and their families than any other healthcare provider. They also interact with all the other members of the healthcare team to collaborate on the needs of the patient (Agency for Healthcare Research and Quality [AHRQ], 2017). Peate et al. (2014) describe the knowledge and skills and standards of competence that student nurses in the United Kingdom must have demonstrated by the time they complete their programs. There are four domains:

1. Professional Values
2. Communication and Interpersonal Skills
3. Nursing Practice and Decision Making
4. Leadership Management and Teamworking (Peate et al., 2014, p. 14)

Nursing school provides students with the strong foundation they will need for their future roles. These domains may be articulated in a different way in different programs, but they should be part and parcel of every nursing program

Paans et al. (2017) conducted a focus group study on what makes an excellent nurse. They completed two phases with a Delphi panel; there were 27 in the first panel, and 26 in the second panel. Based on the results of the focus group and analysis, they identified nine attributes:

1. Analytical
2. Communicative
3. Cooperative

4. Coordinating
5. Disseminate knowledge
6. Empathic
7. Evidence-driven
8. Innovative
9. Introspective

Although this study has limitations, the results can be used to guide curriculum and content and continuing education programs. The Quality and Safety Education for Nurses (QSEN) competencies are also included in the undergraduate and graduate curriculums, with the goal of preparing practitioners who have the knowledge, skills, and attitudes to provide quality of care and promote positive patient outcomes (QSEN, 2021). Curricula must always be updated and reflective of current practice and based on outcomes and evidence. The journey from what Benner (1984) identifies as novice to expert requires a strong foundation and a commitment to lifelong learning.

EDUCATION AND KNOWLEDGE LEVEL AND THEIR RELATION TO SAFETY

A holistic approach to patient safety incorporates multiple approaches; however, education is a vital component and provides foundational and continuing development and competency. The curriculum for undergraduate nursing programs is guided by the various legal and accrediting bodies that inform the curriculum. The undergraduate curriculum prepares nurse generalists and includes content on patient safety, quality of care, and the QSEN competencies. Education level has been correlated with positive patient outcomes.

Many studies have identified a relationship between skill mix, education level, and patient outcomes (AHRQ, 2017). Aiken et al. (2017) describe skill mix as "the percentage of professional nurses among all nursing personnel in the hospital. Total staffing is the total number of all nursing personnel (at all qualification levels) for every 25 patients they cared for" (Aiken et al., 2017). Multiple studies have identified the relationship between increased workloads and inadequate staffing and adverse outcomes, which include infections, falls, and increased length of stay. A lower skill mix, although not as well studied, has also been correlated with an increase in adverse events (Aiken et al., 2002, 2014; Needleman, 2017).

Aiken et al. (2017) conducted a large cross-sectional study in six European countries (Belgium, Finland, Ireland, Spain, Switzerland, England) to determine the association between skill mix and patient outcomes. They defined skill mix as the percentage of professional nurses among all nursing personnel in the hospital. Total staffing is the total number of all nursing personnel (at all qualification levels) for every 25 patients they cared for. They measured the practice environment, doctor–nurse relationships, managerial support, the promotion of quality of care, and managerial support. Nurse education was the percentage of all professional nurses with a bachelor's degree. The practices environment measure is the average score for each hospital across four subscales, indicating (a) managerial support for nursing, (b) nurse participation in hospital affairs, (c) doctor-nurse relations, and (d) promotion of care quality (where a score of 1 would indicate *extremely poor* on all subscales, and a score of 4 would indicate *excellent* on all subscales). Nurse education was calculated as the percentage of all professional nurses in each hospital with bachelor's degrees. They concluded that skill mix was an important indicator, and a greater number of professional nurses was associated with better outcomes for nurses and patients. Conversely, the reduction of skill mix by adding other categories of assistive nursing personnel may decrease safety and quality and may lead to preventable deaths.

There has been a dearth of research to support a more highly educated nursing workforce. Aiken et al. (2017) have been at the forefront of many of the studies which have revealed a correlation with improved patient outcomes. In one study, Aiken found that an increasing the proportion of registered nurses (RNs) with a BS in Nursing by as little as 10% was related to a 7% decrease in patient mortality. The evidence by Aiken and others supported two important initiatives. In 2010, when the Institute of Medicine (IOM) in collaboration with the Robert Wood Johnson Foundation (RWJF, 2009) published the *Future of Nursing* report, several of the initiatives were focused on advanced education and lifelong learning. For example, there was a call to increase the number of baccalaureate-prepared nurses to 80% by 2020. Although there have been increases, this goal has not yet been reached. There was also a call to double the number of doctoral-prepared nurses, encourage lifelong learning, and transition into practice residency programs for undergraduate and graduate nurses (RWJF, 2014). The evidence was compelling, and in 2018, New York state passed a law to require nurses to earn a bachelor's degree in nursing within 10 years of completing an associate degree or diploma nursing program (Newland, 2018). This is not to disparage nurses who are prepared at the associate degree level but to highlight the relevance of a higher educated nursing workforce. Healthcare has become complex and requires nurses to continue to learn and develop critical skills to be more effective practitioners (Newland, 2018). The role and expectations of nurses continue to expand and require a commitment to professional development, competency, and lifelong learning.

Essential Facts

The Institute of Medicine (IOM; 2010) recommends that all new nurses complete a residency program to facilitate their transition into practice.

KEY COMPONENTS OF ORIENTATION

The transition to practice or even to a new unit or role requires a comprehensive orientation. According to the National Council of State Boards of Nurses (NCSBN, 2021), new nurses experience more stress and issues with patient safety than experienced nurses and require orientation and training. The Joint Commission has several standards that guide institutions in creating orientation and competency programs. Although it does not dictate the specific program, it does provide standards and examples to guide the process. The purpose of the orientation is to guide new employees in adjusting and learning about their new organizations, essential job functions, and policies and procedures. There are mandatory topics that must also be included, for example, fire safety, patient safety, infection control, pain management, and sensitivity to cultural diversity (The Joint Commission, 2021). The length of the orientation varies from 6 weeks to 6 months or longer based on the curriculum and required competencies and learning outcomes (Clifford, 2010). Some healthcare institutions have created residency programs to guide the transition into practice. There is a competitive application process, but the program is formalized and may be up to 1 year in duration. There is a combination of didactic classes and a formalized preceptor program. Vizient/American Association of Colleges of Nursing (AACN, 2020) has developed a formalized model of a nurse residency program that has been adopted by myriad healthcare institutions across the country. The program is described as an evidence-based program that focuses on patient outcomes, leadership, and the professional role. It is data-driven with reports of high retention and addresses the IOM's recommendation for formalized nurse residency programs for all new nurses. The benefits include job satisfaction, reduces turnover, improves patient experience, quality of care and safety, and engages more committed caregivers. The NCSBN supports nurse residency programs and has also developed a Transition into Practice Program. The program can be adopted by healthcare institutions and tailored to their needs. There are modules for new nurses and preceptors and the recommended length of the program is 6 months. Unfortunately, not every healthcare institution has the resources to implement residency programs. However, there is a requirement for an orientation program, and many hospitals have staff development specialists who oversee the programs. There is also a plethora of resources that can be used by institutions and individuals. For example, Buettner (2010) published a Essentials book to support the orientation of new emergency room nurses. There are a plethora of conferences and professional organizations that offer valuable resources.

Essential Facts

According to the NCSBN (2021), health institutions with training programs have improved patient outcomes and improved retention rates.

CORE COMPETENCIES RELATING TO SAFE PRACTITIONERS

Competencies are required from the time you enter nursing school and throughout your entire professional career. "Nursing competency includes core abilities that are required for fulfilling one's role as a nurse" (Fukada, 2018, p. 1). Matsutani et al. (2012) described three major components, with seven nursing elements related to them. The first one is the ability to understand people, which requires:

1. Applying knowledge
2. Building intrapersonal relationships

The second one is the ability to provide people-centered care, which requires:

3. Providing nursing care
4. Practicing ethically
5. Collaborating with other professionals

And the third one is the ability to improve nursing quality and includes:

6. Expanding their professional capacity
7. Ensuring the delivery of high-quality nursing

The QSEN competencies as previously discussed require students have the requisite knowledge, skills, and attitudes for the six competencies (Vana et al., 2014; QSEN, 2021):

1. Patient-centered care
2. Teamwork and collaboration
3. Safety
4. Evidence-based practice
5. Quality Improvement
6. Informatics

These competencies incorporate the foundation of care and practice but there are many others that should be included in competency-based programs for nurses. In 2016, the Massachusetts Department of Higher Education revised its core competency program and posits that they emanate from the core of nursing knowledge. In addition to the six QSEN competencies, it includes

- Leadership,
- Communication,
- Professionalism
- Leadership
- Communication
- Professionalism
- Systems-based practice

Clearly, the terminology may differ, but the underlying premise of the competencies is a focus on patient safety, teamwork, ethics, collaboration, evidence, communication, advocacy, and professionalism. It is vital for all nursing programs and healthcare organizations to provide training and education and to develop and measure evidence-based competency programs that are evaluated on an annual basis (Mangold et al., 2018).

IMPORTANCE OF LIFELONG LEARNING

The building blocks of education start with your primary education and continue to develop throughout the years. As a nurse your academic journey begins in your nursing program and that is truly only the beginning. Upon graduation, new nurses are considered what Benner describes as advanced beginners. Some experts believe it takes 10 years in your role to become an expert, but with each transition to a new role, in some ways, you start over again. And even if you achieve the level of expert, with the ever-changing face of healthcare and technology, one must become a lifelong learner (HealthStream, 2017). Indeed, the Future of Nursing report calls for all nurses to be lifelong learners (IOM, 2011). Lifelong learning requires a commitment to ongoing professional development and a commitment to self-motivated personal learning (HealthStream, 2017). There are many ways to engage in lifelong learning. Reading books, articles, and research studies is foundational. Joining professional organizations and attending conferences are other options. Continuing one's formal academic education and participating in your organization's professional development and competency programs should also be part of every nurse's plan for lifelong learning.

SUMMARY

The key attributes of safe practitioners were highlighted in this chapter. These include the following attributes of leadership, advocacy, teamwork, empathic, and being innovative, in addition to skill mix and education level. The significance of a well-planned orientation and residency program was also emphasized in addition to the NCSBN's Transition into Practice model and modules. The relationship between achievement of the competencies and positive patient outcomes were discussed as was the importance of lifelong learning.

VIGNETTE

The turnover rate on the medical-surgical units at a large teaching hospital is 20% among experienced nurses and 50% among new nurses. There is a high rate of falls and pressure ulcers.

Mr. Smallden is a new nurse educator and has been charged with revising the Orientation and Competency Program. What resources should he utilize? Describe the key components of an Orientation and Competency Program. What other measures could be undertaken?

Discussion Questions

1. List three attributes of a safe practitioner.
2. Why are the QSEN competencies, and how do they relate to patient outcomes?
3. What is meant by *skill mix*? Why is it important?
4. Select two of the key initiatives of the *Future of Nursing* report and explain how they relate to patient outcomes.
5. Why is lifelong learning important?

TIPS FROM THE FIELD

A toolkit is available for organizations to offer support to healthcare professionals who make an error. An implementation guide is available to guide healthcare organizations to support their staff to come to terms with the error.

(https://psnet.ahrq.gov/toolkits)

SPECIAL TOPICS

The Patient Safety and Risk Management Unit at the World Health Organization (WHO) created the following agenda:

- Setting global priorities for action developing guidelines and tools
- Providing technical support and building capacity of member states
- Engaging patients and families for safer healthcare
- Monitoring improvements in patient safety
- Conducting research in the area

The WHO (2019) aims to achieve better health outcomes and lower costs, enhance patient experience, and reduce risks and harm.

SUGGESTED CLASSROOM OR UNIT-BASED ASSIGNMENT

A Group Project: Have students or staff work in groups of four to develop a PICOT (patient, intervention, comparison, outcomes, timeframe) on Patient Safety. Each student should select two articles related to the topic to analyze and include in the project.

CASE EXEMPLAR 3.1: REFLECTIONS ON SAFETY AND LIFELONG LEARNING IN NURSING

Elizabeth Riley, DNP, PED-BC, RNC-NIC, CNE

I remember graduating with my BSN degree and thinking, with happiness, that school was finally over. Some of my classmates even burned their lecture notes as a way of closing the chapter. However, I realized very quickly that the learning was not over. The new graduate orientation process was my first glimpse into this phenomenon, with 12 weeks of constant learning about unit policies, procedures, and organizational culture. While formal learning in a classroom was not part of my life anymore, the constant changes to evidence-based practice guidelines, equipment updates, and having to think outside of the box in emergency situations aligned with informal learning to the role. It was then that I realized what my nursing instructors had meant all along about lifelong learning, clinical judgment, and patient safety. Another item that I had not considered was my annual evaluation and RN license renewal, both of which required a set amount of continuing education (CE) hours. I obtained CE hours online from professional nursing organizations and nursing conferences. Once I began looking at the structure of the clinical ladder within my organization, I realized that to move up the ladder required more CE hours, nursing certifications in the specialty, and evidence-based practice projects to enhance nursing care on the unit. As a lifelong learner, all the previously mentioned items are milestones that I have completed during my decade-long career. But not without wise and patient mentors who helped me along the way—find your mentors early on in your career! In telling this story, my main point is that learning in nursing does not end with the commencement ceremony or delivery of the diploma. Learning will be ever constant, occurring every day of your career, to enhance patient safety and clinical practice. The best advice is that planning for this early will greatly aid the transition from a formal learner to a lifelong learner and in turn, promote patient safety.

CASE EXEMPLAR 3.2: REFLECTIONS ON SAFETY AND LIFELONG LEARNING IN NURSING

Fermin Renteria, DNP, APRN, CPNP-PC, CNE

One incident related to safety and lifelong learning that stands out for me happened at my first job after nursing school. I was working on a pediatric hematology-oncology unit before Pyxis machines were used for routine medications, and most medications came to the unit in an envelope with the client's identifying information as well as drug information printed on the outside. In addition, the medication contained in the envelope was labeled with the medication information. One day while gathering and verifying medications, I noticed that one of the liquid oral medications was not the color it normally was. I verified the client's name and drug information on the envelope, verified the drug information on the label attached to the oral syringe, and found that all were accurate. The next step was a call to the pharmacy to ask if the pharmacy had received a new formulation of this particular drug. The pharmacy stated that there was not a new formulation and that the medication contained in the syringe likely was not the correct medication. By being familiar with the appearance of frequently administered medications, not only the drug name, classification, and so on, a medication error was averted, demonstrating the importance of ongoing education and following the six rights of medication administration.

RESOURCES

Hurwitz, B., Hurwitz, B., & Sheikh, A. (2009). *Health care errors and patient safety*. John Wiley & Sons.

Lenburg, C. B., Abdur-Rahman, V. Z., Spencer, T. S., Boyer, S. A., & Klein, C. J. (2011). Implementing the COPA model in nursing education and practice settings: Promoting competence, quality care, and patient safety. *Nursing Education Perspectives*, 32(5), 290–296.

Miscommunication in the OR Leads to Anticoagulation Mishap. (2019). *AORN Journal, 109*(5), 664–666. https://doi.org/10.1002/aom.12660

Res Seifert, P. C. (2012). Implementing AORN recommended practices for transfer of patient care information. *AORN Journal, 96*(5), 475–493. https://doi.org/10.1016/j.aorn.2012.08.011ources

REFERENCES

Agency for Healthcare Research and Quality. (2017). *Nursing and patient safety. A patient safety primer.* https://psnet.ahrq.gov/primer/nursing-and-patient-safety

Aiken, L. H., Clarke, S. P., Sloane, D. M., Sochalski, J., & Silber, J. H. (2002). Hospital nurse staffing and patient mortality, nurse burnout, and job dissatisfaction. *JAMA, 288*, 1987–1993.

Aiken, L. H., Sloane, D. M., Bruyneel, L., Sloane, D. M., Bruyneel, L., Van den Heede, K., Griffiths, P., Busse, R., Diomidous, M., Kinnunen, J., Kózka, M., Lesaffre, E., & McHugh, M. D. (2014). Nurse staffing and education and hospital mortality in nine European countries: A retrospective observational study. *Lancet, 383*, 1824–1830.

Aiken, L. H., Sloane, D., Griffiths, P., Rafferty, A. M., Bruyneel, L., McHugh, M., Maier, C. B., Moreno-Casbas, T., Ball J. E., Ausserhofer, D., & Sermeus. W. (2017). RN4CAST Consortium. Nursing skill mix in European hospitals: cross-sectional study of the association with mortality, patient ratings, and quality of care. *BMJ Qual Saf. 26*(7):559–568. doi: 10.1136/bmjqs-2016-005567

American Association of Colleges of Nursing. (2020). *Vizient/AACN nurse residency program*. https://www.aacnnursing.org/Portals/42/AcademicNursing/NRP/Nurse-Residency-Program.pdf

Benner, P. (1984). *From novice to expert, excellence and power in clinical nursing practice*. Menlo Park, CA: Addison-Wesley Publishing Company.

Buettner, J. R. (2010). *Fast facts for the ER nurse: Emergency room orientation in a nutshell* (2nd ed.). ProQuest Ebook Central. https://ebookcentral.proquest.com

Clifford, T. (2010). Orientation of new nurses. *Journal of Perianesthesia Nursing, 25*(4), 261–262.

Fukada, M. (2018). Nursing competency: Definition, structure and development. *Yonago Acta Medica, 61*(1), 1–7. https://doi.org/10.33160/yam.2018.03.001

HealthStream. (2017). *Lifelong learning in nursing is vital*. https://www.healthstream.com/resources/blog/blog/2017/05/23/lifelong-learning-is-a-vital-effort-for-nurses

Institute of Medicine (US) Committee on the Robert Wood Johnson Foundation Initiative on the Future of Nursing, at the Institute of Medicine. (2011). *The future of nursing: Leading change, advancing health*. Washington (DC): National Academies Press.

Mangold, K., Tyler, B., Velez, L., & Clark, C. (2018). Peer-review competency assessment engages staff and influences patient outcomes. *Journal of Continuing Education in Nursing, 49*(3), 119–126.

Massachusetts Department of Higher Education. (2016). *Massachusetts Nurse of the Future Nursing Core Competencies*. https://www.mass.edu/nahi/documents/NOFRNCompetencies_updated_March2016.pdf

Matsutani, M., Sakyo, Y., Oku, H., Hori, N., Takaya, T., & Miura, Y. (2012). New baccalaureate nursing graduates' perceptions of required nursing competency: An analysis of interview data from nurses in their first year of work. *Seiroka Kango Gakkaishi, 16*, 9–19.

National Council of State Boards of Nursing. (2021). *Transition to practice why transition to practice (TTP)?* https://www.ncsbn.org/transition-to-practice.htm

Needleman, J. (2017). Nursing skill mix and patient outcomes. *BMJ Quality & Safety*, *26*(7), 525–528.

Newland, J. A. (2018). BSN in 10. *The Nurse Practitioner*, *43*(2), 6. https://doi.org/10.1097/01.npr.0000529673.46941.d4

Paans, W., Robbe, P., Wijkamp, I., & Wolfensberger, M. V. (2017). What establishes an excellent nurse? A focus group and Delphi panel approach. *BMC Nursing*, *16*(1), 45.

Peate, I., Wild, K., & Nair, M. (2014). Chapter 1 nursing past, present, and future. In I. Peate, K. Wild, & M. Nair (Ed.), *Nursing practice: Knowledge and care* (pp. 2–23). Wiley.

QSEN. (2021). *Quality and Safety Education for Nurses.* http// qsen.org

Robert Wood Johnson Foundation. (2009). *Unprecedented initiative on the future of nursing launched.* https://www.rwjf.org/en/library/articles-and-news/2009/07/robert-wood-johnson-foundation-institute-of-medicine-launch-unpr.html

Robert Wood Johnson Foundation. (2014). *Building the case for more highly educated nurses.* https://www.rwjf.org/en/library/articles-and-news/2014/04/building-the-case-for-more-highly-educated-nurses.html

The Joint Commission. (2021). *Competency assessment versus orientation.* https://www.jointcommission.org/standards/standard-faqs/office-based-surgery/human-resources-hr/000002152/; https://www.researchgate.net/publication/225271313_Institute_of_Medicine_The_Future_of_Nursing_Report_lifelong_learning_and_certification

Vana, P. K., Vottero, B. A., & Christie-McAuliffe, C. (2014). *Introduction to quality and safety education for nurses: Core competencies (Ch. 1).* Springer Publishing Company.

World Health Organization. (2019). *Patient safety.* https://www.who.int/news-room/fact-sheets/detail/patient-safety

4

Theory-Informed Practice

An ounce of prevention is worth a pound of cure.
—Benjamin Franklin

Nursing is a practice discipline grounded in empirics, aesthetics, knowledge, and evidence. There are many exemplary nursing theorists who influence our education and practice. The nursing theorists highlighted in this chapter inform practice and can be used to develop a culture of safety in our complex healthcare systems.

In this chapter, you will learn:

1. How to utilize Barrett's Power Theory to improve patient outcomes
2. How Watson's Theory of Human Caring Informs a Culture of Safety
3. How to utilize mindfulness and presence
4. How to incorporate Relationship-Based Care (RBC) into your daily practice
5. Ways to practice self-care

THEORY-INFORMED PRACTICE

Every discipline has a set of theories that have been developed to guide its practice. For many years, nursing borrowed theories from other disciplines; however, as more nurses earned advanced degrees, they began to formalize their own body of knowledge. In the 1960s, many theories were borrowed from the disciplines of medicine, sociology, and psychology; however, from the 1980s to the present, there was a paradigm shift, with nurses creating their own theories that included grand theories, middle-range theories, and practice theories. "A theory is a notion or idea that explains experience, interprets observation, describes relationships, and suggests outcomes" (Smith, 2020, p. 7). Nursing theories are used to predict or explain the phenomenon of concern. Nursing's meta-paradigm includes four concepts: the person, the nurse, the environment, and health (Meleis, 1997; Nikfarid et al., 2018; Smith, 2020; Sousa & Hayman, 2002). There are many well-known theorists who have made significant contributions to the discipline of nursing. In this chapter, the contributions of Eileen Barrett and Jean Watson are highlighted with an emphasis on how they can be applied to improve patient outcomes.

ELIZABETH BARRETT'S POWER THEORY

Elizabeth Barrett is a well-known educator, scholar, researcher, and leader with more than 50 years of experience. She studied under Martha Rogers (Science of Unitary Human Beings) and was the first president of the Society of Rogerian Scholars. Barrett's scholarly work revolved around continuing the work of Rogers, which resulted in the development of the Barrett Theory of Knowing Participation in Change and the Power as Knowing Participation in Change Tool (PKPCT). According to Malinski (2018), Barrett (1998, 2010,

Barrett & Caroselli, 1998) derived this theory and related tool during her doctoral program while working with Marta Rogers. Dr. Elizabeth Barrett has a robust website that highlights her background, research, and myriad accomplishments. According to Barrett (2020), evidence supports the fact that human beings have "the power to knowingly participate in change," which can be supported using meditation imagery and therapeutic touch. (https://www.drelizabethbarrett.com/). Health patterning provides a patient with the tools to help patients develop an awareness of the power they hold to participate in change. The individual is guided on how to use their power to take control of their health. Health-patterning modalities use imagery and therapeutic touch to help patients use their power to make lifestyle changes and overcome difficulties in living and struggles with illness (Smith & Gullett, 2020). Power prescriptions are a part of health patterning and are designed to enhance power as freedom and are individualized based on the individual's needs (Smith, 2020, p. 487). Barrett also discusses the power-imagery process. The process uses the PKPCT tool, which guides the health-patterning imagery and power prescriptions. Clearly, many studies have supported the benefits of these interventions, and this author would like to suggest their potential use by patients and healthcare providers in promoting positive patient outcomes. Collaboration among the nursing staff and the patients and family, with a commitment to promoting patient outcomes using health patterning, power prescriptions, and power imagery, could be piloted and evaluated.

JEAN WATSON THEORY OF UNITARY CARING SCIENCE AND THEORY OF HUMAN CARING

The theory of human caring was developed between 1975 and 1979 (Smith & Gullett, 2020). Watson's theory has been expanded and refined throughout the years; however, the basic tenets of caring-healing modalities and nursing as a caring science remain. Watson (2020) sought to provide a balance between curative and carative practices and to provide the discipline of nursing that was grounded in science, philosophical and ethical beliefs and professional standing with itself and the public (Smith, 2020, p. 314). Originally, there were 10 carative factors which are now referred to as caritas. According to Watson (Watson, 2020) "caritas comes from the Latin word meaning to cherish and appreciate, giving special attention to and loving" (p. 315). The 10 caritas in summary follow:

1. Practice of loving-kindness
2. Being authentically present
3. Cultivation of one's own spiritual practices
4. Developing a helping, trusting, authentic caring relationship
5. Authentically listening to another's story
6. Use of self in all ways of knowing
7. Transpersonal genuine teaching–learning experience
8. Creating a healing environment at all levels
9. Assisting with basic needs as a sacred act
10. Opening oneself to spiritual-mysterious existential dimensions of one's own life-death, "allowing for miracles"

Watson's Theory of Caring and Caritas can guide nurses and other healthcare professionals to foster a caring/healing relationship. Watson (2020) describes "transpersonal caring as the gold standard of caring between two people. A healing relationship transcends space and time and is felt by the patient and the nurse". Learning about this and other theories and incorporating a caring/healing philosophy may guide one to create a positive healing environment and promote positive patient outcomes.

KING'S THEORY OF GOAL ATTAINMENT

Imogene King developed the Theory of Goal Attainment (1971). King (1990) posits that the goal of nursing care is to help patients maintain or regain health. In this theory, the nurse and the patient create mutual goals and ways to attain them. This provides the patient with a locus of control with the nurse playing an important role. Patient safety, patient outcomes, and quality improvement measures have been developed and measured using King's mid-range theory of goal attainment. Although the onus of providing safe and effective quality of care is on the nurse, having the patient be actively engaged in their care can promote a positive healing environment.

According to Caceres (2015), King's Theory of Goal Attainment can be used by nurses to improve functional status, which can help promote the well-being and safety of clients. Mutual decision-making between clients/families and nurses may be correlated with improved functional status.

Essential Facts

There are many theories that inform nursing practice with similar concepts and constructs and a focus on patient outcomes.

RELATIONSHIP-BASED CARE

Relationship-Based Care is another way for nurses to promote positive patient outcomes and improve patient outcomes. Relationship-Based Care (RBC) is a philosophy, a framework for aligning values and operations, and an individual way of being (Glembocki & Fitzpatrick, 2013) and evolved from the seminal work of Marie Manthey (2002). The foundation of relationships has 12 basic assumptions that focus on connections, caring, and therapeutic relationships. It requires a commitment by the entire organization to develop a caring and healing environment for all patients. An important component is the three relationships of the nurse, with the self, colleagues, and patient/family's self-care as this is fundamental to helping patients attain optimal health. This model promotes organizational health and improves satisfaction among patients, nurses, physicians, and staff; improves patient outcomes; improves recruitment and retention; and financial health (Glembocki & Fitzpatrick, 2013). Schneider and Fake (2010) posit that RBC improves patient outcomes and can help nurses to develop positive relationships with patients, families, and staff.

UCLA Health uses RBC as an underpinning of its nursing philosophy to promote a caring/healing environment. It is describe as a framework and culture transformation that improves patient satisfaction, safety, quality, and staff satisfaction. Therapeutic relationships with patients and families are integral, and three relationships of the nurse, with the self, colleagues, and the patient/family, are essential for the provision of human and compassionate healthcare (UCLA, n.d.).

The tents and underpinnings of RBC are correlated with many positive outcomes, especially in the areas of quality and patient safety.

MINDFULNESS, PRESENCE, AND SELF-CARE

There are certain buzzwords in nursing that hold important meanings and should be a part of all healthcare providers' vocabulary. As previously discussed, distractions are often associated with adverse events, which lends credence to the practice of mindfulness and being present in the moment so that your lingering presence may be felt by your patients even after you are physically gone. Barbara Dossey (Smith, 2020) discusses mindfulness and presence in relation to her Theory of Integral Nursing. Dossey's theory is complex and incorporates the meta-paradigm of nursing and ways of knowing. According to Dossey (Smith, 2020), mindfulness about intentions, values, and attitudes helps us develop awareness about personal health and promote health on a local and a global level. According to Sibinga and Wu (2010), research supports the use of mindfulness to increase metacognition and improve patient safety. Additional benefits include increased job satisfaction, decreased burnout, and improved mental health and work environment, which may improve clinical decision-making. Graling and Sanchez (2017) suggest that safety management programs in the perioperative area that include mindfulness can help to reduce patient harm and promote a safer environment.

The Ways of Knowing (Carper, 1979) include the fundamental ways of knowing and include empirics (science and evidence), aesthetics (art and true presence), ethics (morals and respect for all), and personal knowing (awareness of self). Munhall (1993) added unknowing (healing presence, mindfulness, authenticity with no preconceptions), and White (1995) added sociopolitical (social, cultural, economic, political, historical) knowing. These are integral to Dossey's theory and to the nurse, and these patterns of knowing guide nurses in bringing their full presence while caring for others. Achieving a state of mindfulness and true presence requires a commitment to self-actualization. Meditation and guided imagery can help one clear one's mind so that they can truly be present in the moment with their patients and families.

The practice of self-care cannot be underscored as it is vital for one's own health and enhances their ability to care for others. Emery (2020), a third-year nursing student, supports the practice of mindfulness and the significance of self-care strategies when caring for others. Self-care has been the subject of numerous studies, nursing theorists, and various nursing organizations. Self-care has been correlated with decreased burnout and turnover, which improves patient safety and outcomes (Hunt, 2015). There are many ways to incorporate health care practices into your life. You can also encourage your patients to engage in self-care practices.

Self-care practices to consider:

- Meditation
- Guided imagery
- Therapeutic touch
- Reiki
- Aromatherapy
- Journaling
- Exercise
- Sports and activities
- Rest and sleep
- Healthy eating
- Walking and hiking
- Reading
- Painting and other crafts

These are just a few examples of self-care practices that you might consider. There are many others, and it is best to develop your own individualized self-care regimen.

SUMMARY

Nursing theories inform practice and can guide nurses in promoting positive patient outcomes. Several theories discussed in this chapter have demonstrated a correlation between patient satisfaction and patient outcomes. RBC has also been shown to improve patient outcomes and organizations; for example, UCLA

Health has adopted this to guide its nursing practice. Mindfulness, presence, and self-care are also correlated with job satisfaction, patient satisfaction, and patient outcomes.

VIGNETTE

Nancy has been asked by her nurse manager to join the Patient Safety Task Force. The task force recommends a pilot using RBC. What steps would Nancy and the task force need to take to design and implement this pilot?

DISCUSSION QUESTIONS

1. Discuss Barrett's power theory and ways to incorporate it into your practice.
2. How can Watson's caritas help nurses create a caring/healing environment?
3. Discuss King's Theory of Goal Attainment?
4. What are the three main relationships in RBC?
5. Discuss the importance of self-care in relation to patient outcomes?

TIPS FROM THE FIELD

Nursing practice should be guided by theory and evidence-based practice. Possessing a spirit of inquiry and asking why something is done is a certain way and how it can be improved are required of all nurses. If your healthcare organization has a research committee, joining it is a good place to start. Collaborating with peers to develop a PICOT project on an area of interest is another way to ensure you are basing your practice on current evidence.

PICOT

P—Patient Population or Problem
I—Intervention
C—Comparison
O—Outcome
T—Timeline

SPECIAL TOPICS: THEORISTS

This chapter provided a brief overview of selected theorists. Many nursing schools and nursing professionals utilize specific theories to define their theoretical framework and philosophical beliefs. The following is a list of well-known theorists you may want to learn more about:

- Jean Watson
- Madeleine Leininger
- Patricia Benner
- Lydia E. Hall
- Joyce Travelbee
- Margaret Newman
- Katharine Kolcaba
- Rosemarie Rizzo Parse
- Ernestine Wiedenbach
- Florence Nightingale
- Hildegard Peplau
- Virginia Henderson
- Fay Abdella
- Ida Jean Orlando
- Dorothy Johnson
- Martha Rogers
- Dorothea Orem
- Imogene King
- Betty Neuman
- Sister Calista Roy—Adaptation theory

SUGGESTED CLASSROOM OR UNIT-BASED ASSIGNMENT

Select a nursing theorist and investigate their theory and applicability to practice. What resonates with you about this theory? How can you use it to inform your practice and promote positive patient outcomes?

CASE EXEMPLAR 4.1: PATIENT SAFETY

Ashley Mulanex

As you read this exemplar consider how one of the theories discussed in this chapter relates to this experience. Which theory might have been applied to this patient situation?

RECEIVING A BRIEF REPORT, PREPARING TO ADMIT A RAPID RESPONSE TEAM ACTIVATION FROM THE FLOOR

A woman in her 90s, with a history of severe aortic stenosis with volume overload and flash pulmonary edema. And a DNR/DNI. We immediately got her on BiPAP and gave her some Lasix. We were able to stabilize her, although it was quite tenuous for a while. Alice (name changed), I learned, was a spirited woman whose aortic stenosis was now at end stage and was not a candidate for surgical or TAVR intervention. She wanted to go home with hospice and be with her family and her dog. As I cared for her over the next several hours, she had multiple episodes of respiratory distress. And while we were able to temporize the situation each time, it seemed clear to me that we were focusing too much on the respiratory distress and less on the cause of her respiratory distress. During those few hours, it became clear that each of these episodes was precipitated by anxiety. Anxiety was not new to Alice; she was a "nervous Nelly" and "wound tight" by nature. As family came to her bedside, she got upset and thrown back into the vicious cycle of acute respiratory distress and flash pulmonary edema, which further exacerbated her anxiety. The likelihood of her going home was diminishing—especially since she loathed BiPAP. As I was charting, I glanced up at her monitor and noticed her heart rate (HR) was 10 BPM faster than it was a few minutes prior. Alice was talking to her family and beginning to get upset again. I quickly entered the room, cranked up the FIO2 on her high flow nasal cannula just as her sat began to drop and hit silence on the monitor. But I wasn't fast enough—she knew she had desatted, and "it was going to happen again." I held her hand and tried to get her to take some deep breaths and calm down, to no avail. Her HR was now tachycardic. She was ramping up again. I grabbed the sides of Alice's face and had a heart-to-heart. "Alice! Look at me. I need you to slow your breathing down. In . . . and out . . . Alice, I know you hate that BiPAP. I need you to breathe with me and try to keep it off, okay? In . . . and out . . . in . . . and out . . ." She needed redirection multiple times, but after a few minutes, her HR returned to baseline, and she began to breathe more easily. No Lasix, no BiPAP, no chaos. I reported off to the night shift nurse that if you watch for it and you get her to control her breathing, you can prevent the whole cycle. I came back the following morning to hear that she had another two episodes of anxiety and pulmonary edema overnight. She had finally tuckered herself out and fallen asleep on the BiPAP. When she woke, she quickly asked to change to the HFNC. I brought up her anxiety to the team during rounds and advocated for a benzodiazepine. The interns initially rebuffed my request, as she was in her 90s and at very high risk for delirium. I countered that her goal was to get home, that her prognosis was so poor that she was expected to pass within the next few days, that she had tolerated them in the past

(I had talked with Alice about what had helped before), and that I was only advocating for something small to "take the edge off." Our palliative care team agreed, and we started her on a low dose of benzo. I kept a close eye on her and went in when I saw her HR start to go up. I'd hold her hand, we'd breathe a few times together, and she'd calm down and continue visiting with her family. I taught her family what I was looking for, how to help redirect her when she gets worked up, and had them breathe with her. We were able to keep her off BiPAP the rest of the shift.

As I reflect on this experience with Alice, I think about how nursing is both heart and science. In my world, the ICU, nursing care is following orders, titrating pressors, administrating antibiotics and other medications, and balancing intake and outputs, but it's also about connecting with others: caring for the person, not the disease. What benefited Alice the most wasn't medical intervention; it was human intervention. It was about connecting with her and focusing on the now and on the breath. It also serves as a wonderful story about how it's far more rewarding when you are responsive to your patients instead of reactive. Responsive is being able to pick up on trends and providing directed intervention. Reactive is waiting until the desat alarm goes off, when her respiratory distress is severe and requires BiPAP, when her HR begins to rise, and her blood pressure starts to drop. Responsive nursing is better not only for our patients but better for nurses too. And Alice? She made it home, after all.

RESOURCES

https://currentnursing.com/nursing_theory/nursing_theorists.html

https://onlinenursing.duq.edu/blog/formulating-a-picot-question

CASE EXEMPLAR 4.2: PATIENT SAFETY

Danielle Walker

The unit council recently noticed a decrease in patient satisfaction scores as well as a decrease in nurse satisfaction. Thinking these two data points may possibly be connected, the council decided to initiate a quality improvement project to improve the care environment and impact quality care and patient satisfaction. After a lengthy discussion and review of the literature, the council decided to use RBC as the foundation for their initiative.

The unit council proposed three unit-based actions aligned with the fundamental concept of the three vital relationships, nurse and patient, nurse and care team, and nurse and self. The actions also aligned with the 12 basic tenets of RBC. First, nurses were encouraged to begin spending a small amount of uninterrupted, focused communication time with patients and their families. While nurses communicate with patients and family all day long, often the time and attention take place while multitasking, providing meds, turning patients, and so on.

Second, the unit began to prioritize nurses actively and intentionally participating in bedside rounds. Nurse participation in bedside rounds, although a goal is often difficult because of systems barriers. While nurses often attend rounds, their participation can be limited by multitasking, being called away for a patient's needs, and unit cultures. Prioritizing focused participation in rounds improves communication among the healthcare team. A key tenet of RBC is the value of every team member and the necessity of connection among team members for synchronized, quality care.

Finally, the council worked with unit management to address staff burnout and frustrations. During daily huddles, nurse concerns and feedback were requested. Managers began to provide unit-wide communication about efforts to confront the issues discussed even when no resolution occurred. Nurses were encouraged to share their feelings about patients and systems within the units and personal and unit achievements and milestones were commemorated as a group.

The intentional acknowledgment of the three relationships in RBC impacted the care environment. Slowly relationships between patients and nurses began to grow. Healthy dialogue developed among members of the care team, leading to healthy, trusting relationships. And nurses began to again feel the positive differences they were making in their workplace and with their patients. These three relationship-based actions led to an improved care environment and patient satisfaction while creating a foundation for transformational change.

RESOURCE

Hedges, C., Nichols, A., & Filoteo, L. (2012). Relationship-based nursing practice: Transitioning to a new care delivery model in maternity units. *Journal of Perinatal & Neonatal Nursing, 26*(1), 27–36.

REFERENCES

Barrett, E. (2010). Power as knowing participation in change: What's new and what's next. *Nursing Science Quarterly, 23*, 47–54.

Barrett, E. A. M. (1998). A Rogerian practice methodology for health patterning. *Nursing Science Quarterly, 11*, 136–138. Google Scholar.

Barrett, E. A. M. (2020). Barrett's Theory of Knowing Participation and Change as cited in M. Smith (Ed.), *Nursing theories and nursing practice* (5th ed.). F. A. Davis Company. https://ebookcentral.proquest.com/lib/adelphi/detail.action?docID=5985004.

Barrett, E. A. M., & Caroselli, C. (1998). A review of the power as knowing participation in change literature. *Nursing Science Quarterly, 11*, 9–16.

Caceres, B. A. (2015). King's theory of goal attainment: Exploring functional status. *Nursing Science Quarterly 28*(2), 151–155. https://doi.org/10.1177/0894318415571601

Carper, B. A. (1979). The Ethics of Caring. *Advances in Nursing Science, 1*(3), 11–20. https://doi.org/10.1097/00012272-197904000-00004

Current Theories. (2020). *Nursing theories.* https://currentnursing.com/nursing_theory

Emery, S. (2020). The importance of self-care for improving student nurse wellbeing. *British Journal of Nursing, 29*(14), 830–830. https://doi.org/10.12968/bjon.2020.29.14.830

Glembocki, M., & Fitzpatrick, J. (2013). *Advancing professional nursing practice: Relationship-based care and the ANA standards of professional nursing practice.* Creative Health Care Management.

Graling, P. R., & Sanchez, J. A. (2017). Learning and mindfulness: Improving perioperative patient safety: Patient safety first. *AORN Journal, 105*(3), 317–321. https://doi.org/10.1016/j.aorn.2017.01.006

Hunt, D. (2014). *The Nurse Professional: Leveraging Your Education for Transition Into Practice* (1st ed.). Springer Publishing Company.

King, I. M. (1990). Health as the Goal for Nursing. *Nursing Science Quarterly, 3*(3), 123–128. https://doi.org/10.1177/089431849000300307

Malinski, V. (2018). The importance of a nursing theoretical framework for nursing practice: Rogers' science of unitary human beings and Barrett's theory of knowing participation in change as exemplars. *Cultura del Cuidado, 15*(2), 6–13. https://doi.org/10.18041/1794-5232/cultrua.2018v15n2.5108

Manthey, M. (2002). *The practice of primary nursing* (2nd ed.). Creative Health Care Management.

Meleis, A. I. (1997). *Theoretical nursing: Development and progress* (3rd ed.). Lippincott.

Munhall, P. L. (1993). 'Unknowing': toward another pattern of knowing in nursing. *Nurs Outlook, 41*(3), 125–128.

Nikfarid, L., Hekmat, N., Vedad, A., & Rajabi, A. (2018). The main nursing metaparadigm concepts in human caring theory and Persian mysticism: A comparative study. *Journal of Medical Ethics and History of Medicine, 11*, 6.

Schneider, M. A., & Fake, P. (2010). Implementing a relationship-based care model on a large orthopaedic/neurosurgical hospital unit. *Orthop Nurs, 29*(6), 374–378. https://doi.org/10.1097/NOR.0b013e3181edd845

Sibinga, E., & Wu, A. (2010). Clinician mindfulness and patient safety. *Journal of the American Medical Association, 304*(22), 2532–2533. https://doi.org/10.1001/jama.2010.1817

Smith, M. (2020). *Nursing theories and nursing practice* (5th ed.). F.A. Davis Company.

Smith, M., & Gullett, D. (2020). Chapter 29 Barrett's theory of power as knowing participation in change. In *Nursing theories and nursing practice* (5th ed.). F.A. Davis Company. https://www.uclahealth.org/nursing/relationship-based-care

Sousa, V., & Hayman, L. (2002). *Nursing theory development.* http://www.objnursing.uff.br/index.php/nursing/article/view/4786/html_393

UCLA. (n.d.). *Relationship-based care.* https://www.uclahealth.org/nursing/relationship-based-care

Watson, J. (2020). Chapter 18: Jean Watson's Theory of Unitary Caring Science and Theory of Human Caring. In *Nursing theories and nursing practice* (5th ed.). F.A. Davis Company.

White, J. (1995). Patterns of knowing: Review, critique, and update. *Advances in Nursing Science, 17*(4), 73–86. https://doi.org/10.1097/00012272-199506000-00007

5

Critical Thinking, Reasoning, Judgment, and Reflection in Nursing Practice

I attribute my success to this: I never gave or took an excuse.

—Florence Nightingale

Critical thinking, reasoning, *and* reflection *are common buzzwords that resonate with healthcare practitioners and educators around the world. The challenge is to understand their meanings and how they inform practice and improve patient outcomes and learn how to develop these important skills. These topics are discussed in this chapter along with the nursing process and how to become a critical listener and reader.*

Clinical judgment is related to critical thinking and is an important component of clinical practice. Nurses and other healthcare providers must make informed decisions in a timely manner when caring for patients. Clinical judgment is something that must be developed and there are various ways to develop this vital skill. Another facet of this is problem-solving and decision-making. These skills are interrelated and are developmental. Everyone is unique, so these skills develop differently.

In this chapter, you will learn:

1. The relationship between critical thinking, reasoning, and reflection
2. Ways to develop critical thinking, reasoning, and reflections
3. Tanner's model for nursing clinical judgment
4. How the nursing process correlates with patient outcome
5. The relationship between clinical judgment and logic and ways to develop these vital skills
6. The Critical Thinking Model for Nursing Judgment

CRITICAL THINKING, REASONING, AND REFLECTION

"Critical thinking and clinical reasoning are known to have a significantly positive correlation with nursing competence" (Chang et al., 2011, as cited in Caputi & Kavanagh, 2018) What is critical thinking? The definition shared by the Foundation of Critical Thinking (2019) is "critical thinking is that mode of thinking—about any subject, content, or problem—in which the thinker improves the quality of his or her thinking by skillfully taking charge of the structures inherent in thinking and imposing intellectual standards upon them" (para. 10). Although this is subject to interpretation and somewhat subjective, a nurse who is a critical thinker has an ability to assess a situation, collect data, think about the possible solutions and potential outcomes, and select the best intervention. "Critical thinking" (CT) is purposeful, self-regulatory judgment that results in interpretation, analysis, evaluation, and inference, as well as explanations of the considerations on which that judgment is based" (Abrami et al., 2015, p. 275). Although there are several concepts and different definitions, some common attributes are required to be a critical thinker. Developing CT is a process that requires knowledge, higher level thinking, inductive and deductive reasoning, assessment, synthesis, and analysis; identifying possible interventions; and selecting the best intervention based on all these aspects (Sullivan, 2012).

According to Sullivan (2012), although CT in the nursing literature was initially discussed in the 1980s, it did not become widely accepted until the 1990s when the "American Philosophical Association's Delphi Research Project outlined a conceptual definition of critical thinking in nursing" (p. 322). CT guides nurses in their problem-solving, decision-making, nursing processes, and clinical judgment, which are required to provide excellent nursing care and promote positive patient outcomes (Sullivan, 2012). Wangensteen et al. (2010) conducted a study on CT dispositions in new nurse graduates in Norway. They concluded that nurse educators and nurse leaders should nurture a desire for learning and curiosity in students and new nurses. Furthermore, nurse educators should be knowledgeable about how foster CT using student-active learning modules. Christianson (2020) posits that nursing students develop CT skills using questioning and probing attitudes. Furthermore, emotional intelligence (EI) is foundational to this process. EI has received significant attention in the literature and reflects an individual's verbal and nonverbal ability to recognize, understand, and manage emotions of self and others. Having a high level of EI is foundational to CT and the ability to cope with the demands and pressures of one's environment, especially in the workplace (O'Boyle et al., 2011). According to Doherty (2009) EI can be developed by working with a mentor, journaling, reflection, and peer feedback. EI is a cognitive skill, and to be successful, one must have cognitive intelligence and EI (Hunt, 2014). Sullivan (2012) posits that educators utilize models such as Paul's model of CT "to teach and assess critical thinking in clinical practice" (p. 324). This model has eight steps that are taught to students to guide them in the development of CT:

1. Purpose
2. Question at issue
3. Information
4. Assumption
5. Implications
6. Concepts
7. Point of view
8. Interpretation (Paul & Elder, 2006)

CT is a process that incorporates the cognitive and affective domains. Nurses need to develop critical thinking skills to provide safe care and promote positive patient outcomes. CT enables nurses to utilize the nursing process to analyze data and determine appropriate interventions (da Costa Carbogim et al., 2017). There are other models and strategies used to help students develop their CT skills. Zandvakili et al. (2019) conducted a study on CT utilizing a novel approach based on "the seven consequences: 'what, when, why, where, who, how and what for' first described by Aristotle in the Nicomachean Ethics" (p. 1). The authors utilized the competency-based 3CA (an acronym for the educational practices of Concept maps, CT, Collaboration, and Assessment) in school-aged children and concluded that this model has merit and needs to be further explored.

CT, reasoning, and reflection are closely intertwined and are foundational to patient outcomes. Assisting nursing students to develop these skills is vitally important. CT requires students and nurses to analyze data. Clinical reasoning requires that one applies reasoning to the situation. Clinical reasoning requires one to possess the attitudes, knowledge, and reflective practice to determine the appropriate course of action for individual patients in specific situations. Clinical judgment (see Chapter 6) requires the student or nurse to intervene appropriately based on the specific situation. In order to provide safe and effective care to all patients, students must develop these three skills in addition to myriad others (Sommers, 2018).

Clinical reasoning is vital for all healthcare professionals. and many decisions must be made quickly which requires competence in this area. Young et al. (2020) completed a mapping of clinical reasoning literature across the professions and concluded that there is a high degree of variability in the clinical reasoning terminology that leads to unclear communication and challenges with operationalizing the concepts. They further posit that their understanding of the concepts will better serve them in the education of their various health professions students. Feili et al. (2018) suggests a holistic approach to teaching clinical reasoning with a balance between self-learning and teaching that focuses on professionalism and clinical reasoning. A pilot study was done with medical students using the show *House* in which medical students watched a part of the show and did other activities, and then students had a critical discussion about the moral and clinical decisions. Feili et al. (2018) posits using media is a good tool to use to develop clinical reasoning, but a conceptual framework should be utilized.

The use of reflection via the use of reflective journaling has been correlated with the development of CT skills. Zori (2016) conducted a descriptive study based on the Delphi study done in 1990 that identified six skills (interpretation, analysis, evaluation, inference, explanation, self-regulation) and seven dispositions (systematicity, analyticity, inquisitiveness, truth seeking, CT confidence, open-mindedness, CT maturity; APA, 1990).

CT has been identified as comprising six skills and seven dispositions. A Delphi study conducted by the APA (1990) included a panel of 46 experts in CT that identified the six skills as interpretation, analysis, evaluation, inference, explanation, and self-regulation (APA, 1990). Zori (2016) conducted a descriptive study on reflective journaling, which was correlated with CT dispositions. She concluded that reflective journaling was a useful tool. Self-reflection and analysis of situations can be quite powerful, and the use of reflective journaling is an excellent way to do so. Self-reflection can help you to become more intentional about your life and is a critical habit that helps you to optimize your performance. Journaling is very personal, and many people keep a journal; however, a self-reflective journal is a bit different. The following may be helpful when incorporating this into your daily life (Wellman, 2019):

- Write down your experiences throughout the day
- Read your entry and reflect on your feelings and insights
- Analyze and create a plan of action for improvement

Wright and Scardaville (2021) completed a review of the literature on reflective journaling and the residency model as a strategy to enhance clinical decision-making and clinical judgment. Reflective practice requires one to examine their practice so that one can improve and grow professionally. Reflective practice helps one develop self-awareness and improve leadership skills and collaboration with other healthcare professionals. They concluded that reflective journaling combined with the nurse residency program helped new nurses engage in self-analysis, develop skills, and enhance knowledge acquisition and self-confidence. Clearly it takes time to learn reflective practice, and journaling is a tool that has been widely recognized to enhance self-reflection, which can improve CT and reasoning skills.

Developing critical listening and reading skills is another important component of enhancing critical thinking and reasoning. Improving listening skills helps students to perform high-level skills such as questioning, associating, sorting, and making conclusions about what they are listening to. Critical reading skills help students develop CT skills by checking the accuracy of information and the appropriateness of evidence (Erkek & Batur, 2020). Processing information is foundational and developmental, and in today's fast-paced high-tech environment, it can be challenging to really listen. That is why communication skills are part and parcel of every nursing program.

NURSING PROCESS

The nursing process is used by nurses to provide holistic patient-focused care and is considered the essential core practice for nurses (*Nursing World*, n.d.). The nursing process has been embraced and widely used across the nursing profession. It provides a systematic way of providing nursing care by following five steps (Alfaro-LeFevre, 2010). The five steps are assessment, diagnosis, planning, implementation, and evaluation. The first step is to assess and gather data. Throughout each step, nurses utilize CT and critical reasoning to determine the most effective goals and interventions (Pokorski et al., 2009).

Assessment is the first step and is considered the data-gathering stage. These data include physiological, psychological, and spiritual assessments in addition to patient history, past history, familial history, social history, head-to-toe assessment, and results of diagnostic tests. The next step is to create a priority nursing diagnosis based on the assessment, which is then used to develop an individualized plan of care. Next, the nurse develops a plan with measurable goals and interventions. The next phase is implementation, during which the nurse provides specific steps for the patient to achieve the goals. The last phase is to evaluate the patient and the effectiveness of the interventions. At this point, the goals are met or the plan is revised based on the status of the patient (*Nursing World,* n.d.). CT, reasoning, and logic guide the entire process.

CRITICAL THINKING MODEL FOR NURSING JUDGMENT

CT and its significant relationship to patient safety have been well established; however, it is still used interchangeably with logic and reasoning, and although there have been models developed, they have not been widely embraced. For example, Kataoka-Yahiro and Saylor (1994) described a CT model for nursing judgment; however, upon reviewing the literature others posit that the nursing process may inhibit a nurse's ability to critically think. The model was adapted from Perry's (1970) mode using "positions" related to CT and developing ethical and intellectual thinking. In the first stage (dualism), the self looks to the authority figure for the correct answers. In the second part (relativism), the self can now detach from the authority figure and can analyze and examine problems. In the third part, (commitment), the self can examine relative merits and alternatives, anticipates choices, and makes personal choices in a relativistic world.

CT dates to Aristotle, and the six main CT questions of "what, when, who, how, why, and where" are considered the mainstay of CT. Zandvakili et al. (2019) conducted a study on the 3CA model. This is a competency-based approach to teaching critical thinking (p. 1). They used the maps and collaboration to help students develop CT skills and concluded that while further research is needed, the use of this model does enhance CT skills.

TANNER'S CLINICAL JUDGEMENT MODEL

Clinical judgment is a required skill for all healthcare professionals (Tanner, 2006). Clinical judgment is related to patient outcomes and, like CT, is developmental. Tanner's (2006) clinical judgment model can be used to help students develop clinical judgment. The model has four stages:

1. Novice stage (clinical situation is perceived)
2. Interpreting stage (understanding the situation)
3. Reflecting stage (focusing on patient's condition and response)
4. Analyzing stage (responding to and considering measures for improved clinical judgment; Yang, 2021; Tanner, 2006)

Yang (2020) conducted a study using Tanner's Clinical Judgment Model and simulation to help new nurses develop clinical judgment. Yang concluded that using Tanner's model during the pre-simulation experience enhanced clinical judgment. Clinical judgment requires the healthcare professional to interpret health problems and use or modify approaches to care based on the needs of the specific patient. Clinical reasoning is a deliberate process that uses evidence to evaluate possible interventions. "Good clinical judgments in nursing require an understanding of not only the pathophysiological and diagnostic aspects of a patient's clinical presentation and disease, but also the illness experience for both the patient and family and their physical, social, and emotional strengths and coping resources" (Tanner, 2006, p. 204).

New nurses are especially weak in the areas of CT, clinical judgment, and reasoning. Nielsen et al. (2016) conducted a study with the Lassater (2007) Clinical Judgment Rubric (LCJR) to provide a framework for preceptors when orienting new nurses. Lassater created this model based on the aspects of Tanner's (2006) model. The Tanner (2006) model and Lassater (2007) rubric form a framework for clinical judgment. "The framework became a starting point for a partnership between practice and academic educators in developing the new hire evaluation process" (Neilsen et al., 2016, p. 85). They concluded that the framework could foster the development of clinical judgment and a foundation for objective evaluation. It's important to continue to conduct research and develop best practices for teaching these critical skills. Recognizing the need to evaluate the new nurse's clinical judgment and decision-making ability, the National Council of State Boards of Nursing (NCSBN, 2021) has developed the NCSBN Clinical Judgment Measurement Model (NCJMM) that has guided the development of the NextGen NCLEX examination.

Essential Facts

Tanner's (2006) Model of Clinical Judgment provides a framework for educators and preceptors to facilitate clinical judgment in nurses.

SUMMARY

There are many factors that affect patient outcomes, and CT, reasoning, and reflection are important skills for all nurses and other healthcare providers to develop and maintain competency. Although these skills are frequently used interchangeably, they are distinct and have different definitions. These skills can be developed and require an ability to critically read and listen. Critical reflection with reflective journaling has been identified as a good way to develop clinical reflection and CT. The nursing process is another factor in the promotion of positive patient outcomes and requires CT and critical reasoning to implement it correctly. Tanner's (2006) Model of Clinical Judgment provides a framework in addition to the LCJR (Lasseter, 2007) . There is consensus on the importance of these skills; however, the best ways to teach and evaluate are still in progress.

VIGNETTE

Nancy is the nurse educator who is working with preceptors and new graduate nurses to guide their orientation. They are using Tanner's (2006) model and Lassater's (2007) rubric. Three of the new nurses are doing well, but two are not. What are some other ways Nancy could help the preceptors and new nurses to improve these vital skills?

Discussion Questions

1. Discuss CT, reasoning, and reflection and compare them.
2. Discuss how to complete a reflective journal and how it is related to patient outcomes.
3. Why is the nursing process important?

4. Describe the key components of Tanner's model?
5. How does Lassater's rubric relate to Tanner's model?

TIPS FROM THE FIELD

Review the four clinical judgment scenarios on the following website . Select one of them and think about the situation. Do you agree with the author's reasoning? What would you do the same or different?

Dupont, S. (2021). *4 "Real World" examples of using clinical judgement to figure out what to do first as a nurse [master post].* https://nursing.com/blog/nursing-clinical-judgement-care-plans

SPECIAL TOPICS: CLINICAL JUDGEMENT MODELS

- Does your school/healthcare institution utilize a clinical judgment model? If so, which one is utilized? Visit the Evolve website (see the following URL) and review the models in the table "Comparison of the Nursing Process with Tanner's Clinical Judgment Model and the NCSBN Clinical Judgment Measurement Model (NCJMM)."
- Think about their similarities and differences. Which one would you recommend for your school or healthcare setting? Why did you select this one? How would you educate your peers on using this model?

https://evolve.elsevier.com/education/expertise/next-generation-nclex/ngn-transitioning-from-the-nursing-process-to-clinical-judgment

SUGGESTED CLASSROOM OR UNIT-BASED ASSIGNMENT

Select a clinical situation that resulted in an error and conduct a root cause analysis? How could the use of a clinical judgment model help prevent this error ?

CASE EXEMPLAR 5.1: HIGH-FIDELITY SIMULATION

Margaret Rosanne Diehl

High-fidelity simulation (HFS) with immediate feedback (e.g., post-simulation debriefing) is an exemplar teaching and learning methodology to foster CT and self-reflection (Gaba, 2004). This is accomplished through experiential learning, a basal characteristic of simulation. HFS fosters a blended type of pedagogical learning incorporating both technical and nontechnical skills (e.g., decision-making, situation awareness, communication, team working, prioritizing, and skill management; Flin et al., 2010). HFS can be defined as an immersive learning experience generally composed of a realistic mannequin connected to computer software producing real-time physiological modeling in which a clinical scenario unfolds and responds to the interventions of the participant(s) (Cannon-Diehl, 2009; Gaba, 2004; Palaganas et al., 2015). Curricula utilizing HFS are constructed so that each simulated scenario incorporates a post-scenario debriefing session. Debriefing sessions often include open, safe discussions regarding participant performance and are extremely valuable for reflection and forming new understanding (Jeffries, 2007; INACSL, 2016).

Simulated curricula can be integrated into almost any learner-centered curricular format for any level of the participant(s) and must be linked to curricular objectives (Gaba, 2003). Simulation depicting physiologic changes allows students to watch cardiovascular and respiratory function change in real time and allows students to intervene. Textbooks and diagrams come alive in a sense and allow CT skills to flow immediately from conceptual knowledge (Gaba, 2004). Simulation has considerable power in providing participants experience with uncommon anatomical or clinical presentations which can be programmed and repeated (Gaba, 2004; Palaganas et al., 2015).

One aspect to consider when developing HFS curricula to enhance critical thinking and reflection is that every scenario should contain both technical and nontechnical components. Technical components can include specific skills, interventions, or tangible activities. Nontechnical components include nontangible type skills such as team working, situation awareness, decision making, and prioritizing/managing tasks, along with communication being involved in all of these (Flin et al., 2010). Technical and nontechnical components are determined as part of scenario design and curricular outcomes desired.

An HFS scenario was designed for graduate nurse anesthesia students to identify, treat, and resolve intraoperative hypotension in a healthy adult patient undergoing a laparoscopic appendectomy. The scenario environment was the nursing simulation laboratory containing a mock operating room. In this scenario, it is helpful if embedded personnel can serve as actors to enhance the fidelity but is not required for students to have a full immersive experience. Student performance expectations were based on their level of clinical education and training. So students who were at the beginning of their clinical rotations experienced milder hemodynamic perturbations and the patient did not worsen. Beginning students were also given more time to solve the hypotension. More experienced students had different expectations, and the scenario unfolded more rapidly with larger decreases in blood pressure. These students were expected to resolve the situation more rapidly.

Post-scenario debriefing provided video playback and highlighted student(s) technical skills (e.g., recognition of hypotension, administration of vasopressors, repeating blood pressure measurements) as well as nontechnical skills (e.g., realizing what aspect of the surgical procedure might be causing the hypotension, communicating with the surgical team, calling for help, resolving hypotension).

Debriefing facilitators often use open-ended questions or comments to obtain student mental frames to help foster accurate self-reflection yielding new understanding. All students participating or watching the scenario are encouraged to offer perspectives and engage in the debriefing sessions. Safe environments are essential for successful debriefs and self-reflection (Rudolph et al., 2006).

High-Fidelity Simulation Development to Foster Critical Thinking and Reflection (Gaba, 2003; Palaganas et al., 2015)

- Curricular objective and simulated activity match (type of knowledge, skill, behavior addressed)
  - Identify the topic to be integrated into the simulation (e.g., hypotension and CT)
- What type of simulation is appropriate (e.g., HFS)?
- Participant characteristics (e.g., student, experienced nurse, number of participants)
  - Participant/student experience level
- Number of participants
- Scenario characteristics
- Age of patient
- Environment
- Details related to scenario unfolding, what is going to happen to reflect or cause the participant to meet the curricular objectives

- Performance expectations or what skills, interventions, and activities will terminate the scenario
- Extent of participant interaction (remote viewing, watching in-person, immersive)
- Method of evaluation/feedback
- Assessment tool (written or verbal, formative or summative)
- Real-time critique as the scenario is unfolding
- Video-based post hoc debriefing session

References

Cannon-Diehl, M. R. (2009). Simulation in healthcare and nursing. *Critical Care Nursing Quarterly, 32*(2), 128–136. https://doi.org/10.1097/CNQ.0b013e3181a27e0f

Flin, R., Patey, R., Glavin, R., & Marin, N. (2010). Anaesthetists' non-technical skills. *British Journal of Anaesthesia, 105*(1), 38–44. https://doi.org/10.1093/bja/aeq134

Gaba, D. M. (2004). The future of simulation in health-care. *Quality and Safety in Health Care, 13*(Suppl. 1), i2–i10. https://doi.org/10.1136/qshc.2004.009878

INACSL Standards Committee. (2016, December). INACSL standards of best practice simulation debriefing. *Clinical Simulation in Nursing, 12*(S), S21–S25. https://doi.org/10.1016/j.ecns.2016.09.008

Jeffries, P. R. (2007). *Simulation in Nursing Education: From Conceptualization to Evaluation*. National League for Nursing.

Palaganas, J. C., Maxworthy, J. C., Epps, C. A., & Mancini, M. E. (2015). *Defining Excellence in Simulation Programs* [Kindle Edition]. Wolters Kluwer Health.

Rudolph, J. W., Simon, R., Dufresne, R. L., & Raemer, D. B. (2006). There is no such thing as nonjudgemental debriefing: A theory and method of debriefing with good judgement. *Simulation in Healthcare, 1*(1), 49–56.

RESOURCES

https://www.ncbi.nlm.nih.gov/pmc/articles/PMC4601210/

https://www.ncsbn.org/14798.htm

Taggart, S., Skylas, K., Brannelly, A., Fairbrother, G., Knapp, M., & Gullick, J. (2021). Using a clinical judgement model to understand the impact of validated pain assessment tools for burn clinicians and adult patients in the ICU: A multi-methods study. *Burns*, *47*(1), 110–126. https://doi.org/10.1016/j.burns.2020.05.032

Yang, F., Wang, Y., Yang, C., Zhou, M. H., Shu, J., Fu, B., & Hu, H. (2019). Improving clinical judgment by simulation: A randomized trial and validation of the Lasater clinical judgment rubric in Chinese. *BMC Medical Education*, *19*(1), 20. https://doi.org/10.1186/s12909-019-1454-9

REFERENCES

Abrami, P. C., Bernard, R. M., Borokhovski, E., Waddington, D. I., Wade, C. A., & Persson, T. (2015). Strategies for teaching students to think critically: A meta-analysis. *Review of Educational Research*, *85*(2), 275–314. https://doi.org/10.3102/0034654314551063

Alfaro-LeFevre, R. (2010). *Applying nursing process: A tool for critical thinking* (7th ed.). Wolters Kluwer Health/Lippincott, Williams & Wilkins.

American Philosophical Association. (1990). *Critical thinking: A statement of expert consensus for purposes of educational assessment and instruction*. Millbrae, CA: The California Academic Press.

Caputi, L. J., & Kavanagh, J. M. (2018). Want your graduates to succeed? Teach them to think. *Nursing Education Perspectives*, *39*(1), 2–3. https://doi.org/10.1097/01.NEP.0000000000000271

Chang, M. J., Chang, Y. J., Kuo, S. H., Yang, Y. H., & Chou, F. H. (2011). Relationship between critical thinking ability and nursing competence in clinical nurses. *Journal of Clinical Nursing*, *20*, 3224–3232. https://doi.org/10.1111/j.1365-2702.2010. 03593.x

Christianson, K. L. (2020). Emotional intelligence and critical thinking in nursing students: Integrative review of literature. *Nurse Educator, 45*(6), E62–E65. https://doi.org/10.1097/NNE.0000000000000801

Defining Critical Thinking. (2021). https://www.criticalthinking.org/pages/defining-critical-thinking/766

da Costa Carbogim, F., de Oliveira, L. B., de Campos, G. G., de Araújo Nunes, E. A., Alves, K. R., & de Araújo Püschel, V. A. (2017). Effectiveness of teaching strategies to improve critical thinking in nurses in clinical practice: A systematic review protocol. *JBI Database of Systematic Reviews and Implementation Reports, 15*(6), 1602–1611. https://doi.org/10.11124/JBISRIR-2016-003035

Doherty, L. (2009). Emotional intelligence vital for patient safety, nurse leaders told. *Nursing Standard, 23*(46), 5. https://doi.org/10.7748/ns.23.46.5.s2

Erkek, G., & Batur, Z. (2020). A comparative study on critical thinking in education: From critical reading attainments to critical listening attainments. *International Journal of Education and Literacy Studies, 8*(1), 142–151. https://doi.org/10.7575/aiac.ijels.v.8n.1p.142

Feili, A., Kojuri, J., & Bazrafcan, L. (2018). A dramatic way to teach clinical reasoning and professionalism. *Medical Education, 52*(11), 1186–1187. https://doi.org/10.1111/medu.13691

Hunt, D. D. (2014). *The nurse professional: Leveraging your education for transition into practice.* Springer Publishing Company.

Kataoka-Yahiro, M., & Saylor, C. (1994). A critical thinking model for nursing judgment. *Journal of Nursing Education, 33*(8), 351–356. https://doi.org/10.3928/0148-4834-19941001-06

Lassater, K. (2007). Clinical judgement dvelopment: Using simulation to create as assessment rubric. *J. Nurs. Educ., 46*(11), 496–503.

Nielsen, A., Lasater, K., & Stock, M. (2016). A framework to support preceptors' evaluation and development of new nurses' clinical judgment. *Nurse Education in Practice, 19*, 84–90. https://doi.org/10.1016/j.nepr.2016.03.012

Nursing World. (n.d.). *What is the Nursing Process?* https://www.nursingworld.org/practice-policy/workforce/what-is-nursing/the-nursing-process/

O'Boyle, E. H., Humphrey, R. H., Pollack, J. M., Hawver, T. H., & Story, P. A. (2011). The relation between emotional intelligence and job performance: A meta-analysis. *Journal of Organizational Behavior, 32*(5), 788–818. https://doi.org/10.1002/job.714

Paul, R., & Elder, L. (2006). *Critical thinking. Tools for taking charge of your learning and your life* (2nd ed.). Pearson Prentice Hall.

Perry, W. G. (1970). *Forms of intellectual and ethical development in the college years: A scheme*. New York: Hold, Rinehart, & Winston.

Pokorski, S., Moraes, M. A., Chiarelli, R., Costanzi, A. P., & Rabelo, E. R. (2009). Nursing process: From literature to practice. What are we actually doing? *Revista Latino-Americana de Enfermagem, 17*(3), 302–307. https://doi.org/10.1590/S0104-11692009000300004

Sommers, C. L. (2018). Measurement of critical thinking, clinical reasoning, and clinical judgment in culturally diverse nursing students – A literature review. *Nurse Education in Practice, 30*, 91–100. https://doi.org/10.1016/j.nepr.2018.04.002

Sullivan, A. (2012). Critical thinking in clinical nurse education: Application of Paul's model of critical thinking. *Nurse Education in Practice, 12*(6), 322–327. https://doi.org/10.1016/j.nepr.2012.03.005

Tanner, C. A. (2006). Thinking like a nurse: A research-based model of clinical judgment in nursing. *Journal of Nursing Education, 45*(6), 204–211. https://doi.org/10.3928/01484834-20060601-04

Wangensteen, S., Johansson, I. S., Björkström, M. E., & Nordström, G. (2010). Critical thinking dispositions among newly graduated nurses. *Journal of Advanced Nursing, 66*(10), 2170–2181. https://doi.org/10.1111/j.1365-2648.2010.05282.x

Wellman, J. (2019). *Benefits of reflective journaling*. Wellman Psychology. https://wellmanpsychology.com/mindbodyblog/2019/8/22/benefits-of-reflective-journaling

Wright, J., & Scardaville, D. (2021). A nursing residency program: A window into clinical judgement and clinical decision making. *Nurse Education in Practice, 50.* http://dx.doi.org.libproxy.adelphi.edu/10.1016/j.nepr.2020.102931

Yang, S. (2021). Effectiveness of neonatal emergency nursing education through simulation training: Flipped learning based on Tanner's Clinical Judgement Model. *Nursing Open*, *8*(3), 1314–1324. https://doi.org/10.1002/nop2.748

Young, M. E., Thomas, A., Lubarsky, S., Gordon, D., Gruppen, L. D., Rencic, J., Ballard, T., Holmboe, E., Da Silva, A., Ratcliffe, T., Schuwirth, L., Dory, V., & Durning, S. J. (2020). Mapping clinical reasoning literature across the health professions: A scoping review. *BMC Medical Education*, *20*(1), 107. https://doi.org/10.1186/s12909-020-02012-9

Zandvakili, E., Washington, E., Gordon, E. W., Wells, C., & Mangaliso, M. (2019). Teaching patterns of critical thinking: The 3CA model—Concept maps, critical thinking, collaboration, and assessment. *SAGE Open*, *9*(4). https://doi.org/10.1177/2158244019885142

Zori, S. (2016). Teaching critical thinking using reflective journaling in a nursing fellowship program. *Journal of Continuing Education in Nursing*, *47*(7), 321–329. https://doi.org/10.3928/00220124-20160616-09

6

Prioritization and Delegation in Nursing Practice

The very first requirement in a hospital is that it should do the sick no harm.

—Florence Nightingale

Prioritization requires nurses to make serious decisions about patients and patient care. Prioritization requires nurses to utilize the ABCs (airway, breathing, circulation), Maslow's hierarchy of needs, ranking of patient risk, knowledge of time-sensitive indicators, and interpretation of patient data. New graduate nurses may find this particularly challenging. Strategies to help new nurses develop prioritization skills include teaching students about risk potential and ways to identify patients at highest risk. They should also be given opportunities to practice prioritizing patient care (Jessee, 2019). Routinization and standardization are correlated with improved healthcare (Rusjan & Kiauta, 2019). Standardizing care and interventions have the potential to improve patient safety. The World Health Organization (WHO) created the High 5s project, which is a global patient safety initiative. The overarching goal is to achieve measurable, sustainable, and significant improvements in patient safety through the development of standard operating protocols. To date, evidence has been strong, but further development and evaluation are needed (Leotsakos et al., 2014). The Agency for Health Care Research and Quality (AHRQ, 2021) Surveys on Patient Culture began in 2001 to guide healthcare organizations in assessing staff's perception of a culture of safety.

Delegation is another key aspect of the nurse's role and is directly correlated with improved patient safety. Staff nurses must learn how to effectively delegate in a timely manner to unlicensed assistive personnel. Scope of practice is the underpinning of delegation as one must know what can be delegated based on the role and responsibilities of the team members. The nurse must also verify that tasks that have been delegated have been completed correctly.

In this chapter, you will learn:

1. Prioritization (description, significance, and ways to develop)
2. Routinization and standardization
3. Intuition and perception
4. Ethics of nursing
5. Delegation (description, significance, ways to develop)
6. How to become an effective delegator
7. Understanding what to delegate
8. Scope of practice

PRIORITIZATION

Prioritizing patient care takes time and practice. Benner's (1982) novice to expert model demonstrates the developmental process of transitioning through the stages. According to Caputi (2018), prioritization is a learned skill, and in order to produce proficiency, there needs to be deliberate work in school that focuses on this. Nursing students must be able to prioritize data, sift through clues and determine the most appropriate intervention (Eisenmann, 2021). There is a constant need to assess the individual patient and the overall patient assignment as there will always be competing demands. One approach to teaching students prioritization is the "Who, What, & Why?" exercise. Clinical education theory guided this approach to clinical education. Students must be given meaningful feedback during clinical and consistent use of "Who, What, Why" allows students to practice prioritization in addition to improving metacognition and collaborative discourse with peers (Jessee, 2019).

Prioritization is something that is learned in nursing school and must continue to be developed throughout one's nursing career. There will always be competing demands and when caring for multiple patients one must always think about their assignment and determine which patients and/or assessments and procedures should be done first. Patient acuity and current status should always be considered when prioritizing care. Dupont (2021) recommends that after receiving a report, the nurse should create a "to-do list" and start with the ABCs. The next step is to develop the non-urgent tasks that need to be done. Time management, organization, and delegation are also required to guide the prioritization process. Certainly, there are guidelines and recommendations; however, it is important to utilize the knowledge, skills, and theories to develop your individualized approach to prioritization.

ROUTINIZATION AND STANDARDIZATION

The significance of standardization and routinization in relation to patient safety has been discussed in the literature. Standardization of care requires a process that is based on best practices and coordination of care. Process standardization is correlated with improved communication and decreases process errors (Rusjan & Kiatu, 2019). Standardization of care includes clinical protocols that may be adopted by various healthcare organizations and incorporated into their policy and procedures. Not everyone believes that standardization should be implemented. For example, Petrakaki and Kornelakis (2016) discuss the disconnect between technology, standardization, and autonomy. They posit that in high-skilled roles, there needs to be an integration of autonomy with the standardization of care and the use of technology. There may be some areas that are more conducive to standardization. Malekzadeh et al. (2013) conducted a study on a standardized shift handover protocol in ICUs and found that it improved patient safety in the area of basic nursing care and continuity of care. As previously stated, communication issues are directly correlated with many patient errors, and the change of shift is a critical time with no room for errors.

According to Simon et al. (2016), routinization is a process in which activities are developed and should be followed in the same way. This is considered the journey, and when these activities become institutionalized, they improve patient safety. Routinization is correlated with standardization, where something may become second nature when it is part of a routine. Collinsworth et al. (2021) conducted a study on routinization and the

ABCDE bundle in ICUs. "The ABCDE (Awakening and Breathing Coordination, Delirium monitoring and management, and Early exercise/mobility) bundle has been associated with reductions in delirium incidence and improved patient outcomes but has not been widely adopted" (p. 333). Collinsworth et al. (2021) conducted a study on the routinization and implementation of the ABCDE bundle and concluded that increased routinization was correlated with adherence to the steps in the bundle and improved patient outcomes. Routinization has been studied in the integration of evidence-based practice, which has been correlated with improved patient outcomes and patient safety (Renolen et al., 2019).

INTUITION AND PERCEPTION

Intuition is defined as "a natural ability or power that makes it possible to know something without any proof or evidence" (Merriam-Webster, 2021). Sometimes we follow our intuition, and other times we question it. Many nurses, especially experienced ones, have developed a strong intuition about their patients, and interestingly the literature recognizes the significance of the "nursing intuition" (Melin-Johannson et al., 2017). Four Seasons Health Care (FSHC) head of nursing Joanne Strain has urged nurses to use their "nursing intuition" when getting to know a person during assessments. Intuition has been described as insight or a way of knowing without using rational thinking. It is also considered legitimate nursing knowledge and is supported by Benner. Although intuition is thought to be related to patient outcomes there is a lack of evidence to support it (Hassani et al., 2016). Melin-Johannson et al. (2017) posit that intuition is a process based on knowledge and is more than a "gut feeling." They suggest that nurses should use intuition to support decision-making, which can promote patient safety. Intuition in clinical decision-making is correlated with patient safety and patient outcomes (Holm & Severnsson, 2016). Nurse practitioners use intuition as a way of knowing in clinical practice. "Even if clinical experience is found to increase the use of intuition, the question remains if the use of intuition leads to more accurate clinical decisions" (Rosciano et al., 2016, p. 565). Nursing intuition can play an important role in patient safety; however, due to a paucity of evidence, further study is warranted.

The perception of nurses in various areas has been examined, including the perception of patient safety and patient outcomes. One study found that on the unit-level ICU nurses had a positive perception of patient safety (Sidani et al., 2016; Ballangrud et al., 2012). Top and Tekingündüz (2015) found that nurses in acute and rehab settings may not have a positive perception of EBP and patient outcomes due to their limited applicability across practice settings. They posit that further exploration is warranted. Some experts suggest that the perception of patient safety should be cultivated in nurses as it is correlated with patient outcomes and should be viewed as a continuous process. The perception of nurses and patient safety was the subject of a study by Skagerström et al. (2017), who examined nurses' perceptions, attitudes, and beliefs of involving patients in patient safety. Nurses' perceptions of the significance of involving patients in their care are correlated with patient outcomes. Conversely, a poor perception of patient safety culture has been correlated with an increased rate of infections, a poor work environment, negative outcomes, and increased mortality (Forbes et al., 2020). Perceptions among new graduate nurses and experienced nurses were studied by Forbes et al. (2020), who found that new graduate nurses had a more positive perception of patient safety culture, which was the most significant 24 months postgraduation. They found similarities in perceptions regarding communication and the greatest difference in how managers responded to mistakes. This may lead to increased burnout, and they recommend that educators focus more on this area with increased education, debriefing, and further study. The perception of health care has been examined from the patient's perspective too. Patients may detect mishaps related to the coordination of their care and be alerted to the possibility of a lack of care by their providers (Hincapie et al., 2016). Perception is subjective; however, there is some correlation between perception and patient outcomes.

ETHICS

Nurses have an ethical, legal, and moral obligation to provide quality care and promote positive patient outcomes. Ethical principles are applied across disciplines. The nursing profession (Benbow, 2017) has a Code of Ethics and International Code of Ethics that should be used to guide their practice. Ethical values guide the practitioner in identifying intentions, motives, and actions that are valued and govern the moral behavior of conduct (Epstein & Turner, 2015). Ethical values and practice are two of the vital foundations of nursing practice. Nurses deal with ethical dilemmas that may arise at any given time and must be knowledgeable about the ethical principles and how they should inform their care and practice (Haddad & Geiger, 2021).

The four main ethical principles are as follows:

1. Beneficence (to do good)
2. Nonmaleficence (avoid harm)
3. Autonomy (patient's right to self-determination)
4. Justice (fair and ethical treatment)

These principles should guide healthcare providers in the care and management of patients. Moral obligations require one to do what is right based on legal and ethical principles (Varkey, 2021). Ethical patient safety guides the management of nursing care, the implementation of ethical protocols, and the protection of human dignity (Kangasniemi et al., 2013). These principles must become ingrained and serve as the foundation for becoming a safe and ethical practitioner who will strive to use and apply the knowledge, skills, and attitudes necessary for providing quality of care and promoting positive outcomes.

Essential Facts

Ethics within healthcare are important because workers must recognize healthcare dilemmas and make good judgments and decisions based on their values while keeping within the laws that govern them. To practice competently with integrity, nurses, like all healthcare professionals, must have regulation and guidance within the profession. The American Nurses Association (ANA) has developed the Code of Ethics for this purpose (Haddad & Geiger, 2021).

DELEGATION AND SCOPE OF PRACTICE

The art of delegation is a developmental process and can be challenging, especially for new nurses. It's important to learn what can be delegated. Delegation must be based on the scope of practice and experience level of the nurse or healthcare provider. Oftentimes, registered nurses delegate tasks to unlicensed assistive personnel. An understanding of the practice role and clear communication are required. It is also important to follow the specific policies and procedures of the specific healthcare organization. Young et al. (2016) conducted a study on nurse delegation to unlicensed assistive personnel in community-based settings in New Jersey. "States vary in their implementation of nurse delegation, with different patterns of adoption, interpretation of RN role and accountability, and expectations for training (Reinhard et al., 2006; Young & Siegel, 2016, as cited in Young et al., 2017, p. 7). In the study, several tasks were delegated to the unlicensed personnel:

- Medication administration
- Wound care
- Glucometer readings
- Catherization

Based on the positive results of the study and reviews by several agencies, the New Jersey Board of Nursing adopted a new policy to allow nurses to delegate tasks to unlicensed personnel.

Wagner (2018) found that nurses tended to delay the decision to delegate but that effective communication and delegation correlated with patient satisfaction and decreased patient falls. Patients must be assessed thoroughly prior to delegating clinical tasks to unlicensed assistive personnel (Snowdon et al., 2020). The ANA (2012) created a resource to guide registered nurses in the process of delegation. The resource includes a very helpful decision tree (see resource list).

Essential Facts

RNs often delegate nursing tasks to other team members. RNs within the healthcare team are accountable for determining the level of supervision needed and for supervising those to whom they have delegated tasks. RNs are accountable for the decision to delegate and for the adequacy of nursing care provided to the healthcare consumer (ANA, 2012).

RNs must know their scope of practice and the scope of practice of anyone to whom they will delegate tasks.

Each state has a similar yet distinct scope of practice, so it is important to know one's specific scope. Only RNs can assess, but licensed practical nurses may administer treatments and medications. The scope of practice for RNs varies by state.

In New York state, our rights and responsibilities as nurses are defined by the Nurse Practice Act (State Education Law, Article 139): The practice of the profession of nursing as a registered professional nurse is defined as

> diagnosing and treating human responses to actual or potential health problems through such services as case finding, health teaching, health counseling, and provision of care supportive to or restorative of life and well-being, and executing medical regimens prescribed by a licensed physician, dentist or other licensed health care provider legally authorized under this title and in accordance with the commissioner's regulations.

It is important to review your state's or country's nurse practice act and be sure to practice within the guidelines.

The scope of practice of nursing assistants includes nine tasks:

1. Personal care skills
2. Safety/emergency procedures
3. Infection control
4. Basic nursing skills
5. Communication and interpersonal skills
6. Care of cognitively impaired residents
7. Basic restorative care
8. Residents' rights
9. Mental health and social needs (McMullen et al., 2015)

It is important for RNs to remember that part of delegation is supervision and ensuring that the task has been done as per the policies of the healthcare organization. Being an effective delegator also requires clear communication and realistic expectations based on the individual's level of experience and demonstrated competency in their role.

SUMMARY

Healthcare has become increasingly complex and requires nurses to possess the knowledge, skills, and attitudes to provide quality care. Nursing intuition has been discussed in the literature, and although further study is needed, it is correlated with patient outcomes. Standardization and routinization may play a role in patient outcomes. Delegation is an important responsibility of the registered nurse and must be done based on scope of practice, experience, and competency level.

VIGNETTE

Miranda is a new nurse and having a difficult time prioritizing care. As the nurse educator, how would you help her in developing these skills?

Discussion Questions

1. Discuss your views of nursing intuition.
2. What is the relationship between standardization and patient safety?
3. What are ways to prioritize patient care?
4. List and describe ethical principles and how they inform nursing practice.
5. Discuss delegation and ways to delegate effectively.

TIPS FROM THE FIELD

The ANA Principles for Practice for Delegation by Registered Nurses to Unlicensed Assistive Personnel is a good resource for learning more about delegation and includes a very helpful delegation chart (www.nursingworld.org/~4af4f2/globalassets/docs/ana/ethics/principlesofdelegation.pdf).

SPECIAL TOPICS: ETHICS

Knowledge of ethical principles is required of all nurses and must advocate for their patients. Most healthcare organizations have an ethics committee, and it is important to know when an issue should be presented to them (Haddad & Geiger, 2021).

According to Avant Healthcare Professionals (2021), the top five ethical dilemmas faced by nurses include the following:

- Informed consent
- Protecting patient privacy and Confidentiality
- Shared patient decision-making,
- Addressing advanced care planning
- Inadequate resources and staffing

SUGGESTED CLASSROOM OR UNIT-BASED ASSIGNMENT

Look up your state's or province's nurse practice act and compare and contrast the similarities and differences to two other state's or province's practice acts? Discuss the similarities and differences.

RESOURCES

https://avanthealthcare.com/blog/ethical-issues-in-nursing.stml

www.ncbi.nlm.nih.gov/books/NBK526054

www.nursingworld.org/~4af4f2/globalassets/docs/ana/ethics/principlesofdelegation.pdf www.myamericannurse.com/ethical-issues-in-healthcare

www.oacbdd.org/clientuploads/Docs/2014/Convention/Session%20302%20(Deb%20Maloy).pdf

REFERENCES

Agency for Healthcare Research and Quality. (2021). *About SOPS*. https://www.ahrq.gov/sops/about/index.html

American Nursing Association. (2012). *ANA's principles of delegation for registered nurses to unlicensed assistive personnel*. https://www.nursingworld.org/~4af4f2/globalassets/docs/ana/ethics/principlesofdelegation.pdf; https://www.nursingworld.org/practice-policy/scope-of-practice/

Avant Healthcare Professionals. (2021, September 8). Top 5 ethical issues in nursing. Blog. https://avanthealthcare.com/blog/ethical-issues-in-nursing.stml

Ballangrud, R., Hedelin, B., & Hall-Lord, M. (2012). Nurses' perceptions of patient safety climate in intensive care units: A cross-sectional study. *Intensive & Critical Care Nursing, 28*(6), 344–354. https://doi.org/10.1016/j.iccn.2012.01.001

Benbow, M. (2017). Law and ethics in nursing and healthcare: An introduction (2nd ed.). *Nursing Standard, 31*(31), 34–34. https://doi.org/10.7748/ns.31.31.34.s38

Benner, P. (1982). From novice to expert. *American Journal of Nursing, 82*(3), 402–407.

Caputi, L. (2018). *Think like a nurse: A handbook*. Windy City Publishing.

Collinsworth, A. W., Brown, R., Cole, A. L., Jungeblut, C., Kouznetsova, M., Qiu, T., Richter, K. M., Smith, S., Masica, A. L. (2021). MSCI implementation and routinization of the ABCDE bundle. *Dimensions of Critical Care Nursing, 40*(6), 333–344. https://doi.org/10.1097/DCC.0000000000000495

Dupont, S. (2021). *How to prioritize nursing care*. https://nursing.com/blog/prioritize-nursing-tasks/

Eisenmann, N. (2021). An innovative clinical concept map to promote clinical judgment in nursing students.

Journal of Nursing Education, 60(3), 143–149. https://doi.org/10.3928/01484834-20210222-04

Epstein, B., & Turner, M. (2015). The nursing code of ethics: Its value, its history. *Online Journal of Issues in Nursing, 20*(2), 4.

Forbes, T. H., Scott, E. S., & Swanson, M. (2020). New graduate nurses' perceptions of patient safety: Describing and comparing responses with experienced nurses. *Journal of Continuing Education in Nursing, 51*(7), 309–315. https://doi.org/10.3928/00220124-20200611-06

Haddad, L., & Geiger, R. (2021). *Nursing ethical considerations*. National Library of Medicine: National Center for Biotechnology Information. https://www.ncbi.nlm.nih.gov/books/NBK526054/

Hassani, P., Abdi, A., & Jalali, R. (2016). State of science, "Intuition in Nursing Practice": A systematic review study. *Journal of Clinical and Diagnostic Research, 10*(2), JE07–JE11. https://doi.org/10.7860/JCDR/2016/17385.7260

Hincapie, A. L., Slack, M., Malone, D. C., MacKinnon, N. J., & Warholak, T. L. (2016). Relationship between patients' perceptions of care quality and health care errors in 11 countries. *Quality Management in Health Care, 25*(1), 13–21. https://doi.org/10.1097/QMH.0000000000000079

Holm, A. L., & Severinsson, E. (2016) A systematic review of intuition—A way of knowing in clinical nursing? *Open Journal of Nursing, 6*, 412–425. https://doi.org/10.4236/ojn.2016.65043

Jessee, M. A. (2019). Teaching prioritization: "who, what, & why?". *Journal of Nursing Education, 58*(5), 302–305. http://dx.doi.org.libproxy.adelphi.edu/10.3928/01484834-20190422-10

Kangasniemi, M., Vaismoradi, M., Jasper, M., & Turunen, H. (2013). Ethical issues in patient safety: Implications for nursing management. *Nursing Ethics, 20*(8), 904–916. https://doi.org/10.1177/0969733013484488

Leotsakos, A., Zheng, H., Croteau, R., Loeb, J. M., Sherman, H., Hoffman, C., Morganstein, L., O'leary, D., Bruneau, C., Lee, P., & Duguid, M. (2014). Standardization in patient safety: The WHO high 5s project. *International Journal for Quality in Health Care*. https://pubmed.ncbi.nlm.nih.gov/24713313/

Malekzadeh, J., Mazluom, S. R., Etezadi, T., & Tasseri, A. (2013). A standardized shift handover protocol: Improving nurses' safe practice in intensive care units. *Journal of Caring Sciences*, *2*(3), 177–185. https://doi.org/10.5681/jcs.2013.022. https://www.merriam-webster.com/dictionary/intuition

McMullen, T. L., Resnick, B., Chin-Hansen, J., Geiger-Brown, J. M., Miller, N., & Rubenstein, R. (2015). Certified Nurse Aide scope of practice: State-by-state differences in allowable delegated activities. *J Am Med Dir Assoc*, *16*(1), 20–24. https://doi.org/10.1016/j.jamda.2014.07.003.

Melin-Johansson, C., Palmqvist, R., & Rönnberg, L. (2017). Clinical intuition in the nursing process and decision-making—A mixed-studies review. *Journal of Clinical Nursing*, *26*(23-24), 3936–3949. doi: 10.1111/jocn.13814. Epub 2017 Jun 22.

Merriam-Webster. (2021). *Dictionary*. The Merriam-Webster. Com Dictionary. https://www.merriam-webster.com/

Petrakaki, D., & Kornelakis, A. (2016). "We can only request what's in our protocol": Technology and work autonomy in healthcare. *New Technology, Work & Employment*, *31*(3), 223–237. https://doi-org.libproxy.adelphi.edu/10.1111/ntwe.12072

Reinhard, S. C., Young, H., Kane, R. A., & Quinn, W. V. (2006). Nurse delegation of medication administration for elders in assisted living. *Nursing Outlook*, *54*, 74–80.

Renolen, Å., Hjaelmhult, E., Høye, S., Danbolt, L. J., & Kirkevold, M. (2019). Creating room for evidence-based practice: Leader behavior in hospital wards. *Research in Nursing & Health*, *43*(1), pp. 90–102. https://doi.org/10.1002/nur.21981

Rosciano, A., Lindell, D., Bryer, J., & DiMarco, M. (2016). Nurse practitioners' use of intuition. *Journal for Nurse Practitioners*, *12*(8), 560–565. http://dx.doi.org/10.1016/j.nurpra.2016.06.007

Rusjan, B., & Kiauta, M. (2019). Improving healthcare through process standardization: A general hospital case study. *International Journal of Health Care Quality Assurance*, *32*(2), 459–469. http://dx.doi.org.libproxy.adelphi.edu/10.1108/IJHCQA-06-2018-0142

Sidani, S., Manojlovich, M., Doran, D., Fox, M., Covell, C. L., Kelly, H., Jeffs, L., & McAllister, M. (2016). Nurses' perceptions of interventions for the management of patient-oriented outcomes: A key factor for evidence-based practice. *Worldviews on Evidence-Based Nursing, 13*(1), 66–74. https://doi-org.libproxy.adelphi.edu/10.1111/wvn.12129

Simon, M., McGuire, R., Lynch, H., Moodey, K., Edmonds, A., Moore, E., & Jordan, H. (2016). The journey toward routinization: Triage nursing and the success of an emergency department-based routine HIV testing program: JEN. *Journal of Emergency Nursing, 42*(2), 183–185. http://dx.doi.org/10.1016/j.jen.2016.02.003

Skagerström, J., Ericsson, C., Nilsen, P., Ekstedt, M., & Schildmeijer, K. (2017). Patient involvement for improved patient safety: A qualitative study of nurses' perceptions and experiences. *Nursing Open, 4*(4), 230–239. http://dx.doi.org/10.1002/nop2.89

Snowdon, D. A., Storr, B., Davis, A., Taylor, N. F., & Williams, C. M. (2020). The effect of delegation of therapy to allied health assistants on patient and organisational outcomes: A systematic review and meta-analysis. *BMC Health Services Research, 20*(1), 491–491. https://doi.org/10.1186/s12913-020-05312-4

Top, M., & Tekingündüz, S. (2015). Patient safety culture in a Turkish public hospital: A study of nurses' perceptions about patient safety. *Systemic Practice and Action Research, 28*(2), 87–110. http://dx.doi.org/10.1007/s11213-014-9320-5

Varkey, B. (2021). Principles of clinical ethics and their application to practice. *Medical Principles and Practice, 30*, 17–28. https://doi.org/10.1159/000509119

Wagner, E. A. (2018). Improving patient care outcomes through better delegation-communication between nurses and assistive personnel. *Journal of Nursing Care Quality, 33*(2), 187–193. https://doi.org/10.1097/NCQ.0000000000000028

Young, H. M., & Siegel, E. O. (2016). The right person at the right time: Ensuring person centered care. *Generations, 40*, 47–55.

Young, H. M., Farnham, J., & Reinhard, S. C. (2016). Nurse delegation in home care: Research guiding policy change. *Journal of Gerontological Nursing, 42*(9), 7–15. http://dx.doi.org/10.3928/00989134-20160811-04.

7

Leadership Skills and Patient Outcomes in Nursing Practice

It takes leadership to improve safety.

—Jackie Stewart

The significance of the role of the nurse leader in nursing and healthcare organizations has been well documented. There are many leadership theories and styles and while some believe that leaders are born which may be true many leaders need education and mentoring. Leadership has been defined by George and Jones (2005) as "the exercise of influence by one member of a group or organization over other members to help the group or organization achieve its goals" (p. 375). In healthcare organizations leadership occurs at multiple levels and requires leaders that are knowledgeable, fair, and balanced. The nurse leader on the unit level and the organization level plays a significant role in the culture of the organization, especially in patient care and practice. Leadership styles vary among leaders and situations, but the preferred leadership style in nursing is one that is transformational. In more recent times, emotional intelligence has become a significant attribute of exemplary leaders.

In this chapter, you will learn:

1. Leadership theory
2. Leadership styles and development
3. Role of the nurse leader throughout the patient care process
4. Emotional intelligence
5. Critical thinking and emotional intelligence

LEADERSHIP

Leadership theories have evolved from behavioral in nature starting with the "great man" theory to the current ones that are more focused on the relationship of the leader and the follower (Hunt, 2012). According to Bass and Bass (2008) current leadership theories focus on interpersonal dynamics in lieu of managerial tasks and leader–follower exchanges. According to Benmira and Agboola (2021), leadership is complex, and despite being studied extensively throughout the years, it is still the subject of much debate. "Bennis notes that 'leadership is the most studied and least understood topic of any in the social sciences' and 'never have so many laboured so long to say so little'" (Bennis, 2009, as cited in Benmira & Agboola, 2021, p. 3). The earliest recorded theory is the great man theory (1840). The core belief is that leaders are born, not made (Benmira & Agboola, 2021), and was based on the notion that leadership qualities were inherent in some people, and this influenced why they became leaders. They were viewed as exceptional people, and within this theory, "to be good leaders, they had to be male" (Bolden et al., 2003, as cited in Hunt, 2012, p. 55). The trait theories evolved from this theory and posited that leaders could be made or born (Buchanan & Huczynski, 2017). Most leader traits can be organized into three categories: interpersonal attributes, demographics, and traits related to task competence (Derue et al., 2011). Behavioral theory followed and is still the foundation for many leadership development programs (Benmira & Agboola, 2021). "Behaviorist" theories described the action a leader takes and involved either consideration or initiating structure (George & Jones, 2005). The third dimension, Decision-Centralization, is the extent to which a leader allows their subordinates to participate in decision-making (Yukl, 1971). Following this theory was the work of Fielder (1967), who described situational leadership, in which the style of leadership matches the situation. However, he posited that matching the leader to the situation might be more effective (Fiedler & Chemers, 1974; Bolden et al., 2003 as cited in Hunt, 2012). Transactional leadership is based on an exchange of rewards and punishment of the followers. According to Vecchio et al. (2008), transactional leadership utilizes rewards with subordinates to exert influence over their subordinates so that they complete their tasks as required.

Transactional theory or leader–member exchange (LMX) theory posits that each relationship between the leader and member is unique and that "dyads" are formed where the leader and member help each other (George & Jones, 2005). LMX theory has been correlated with positive outcomes of job satisfaction, commitment, and job performance of the followers (Gutermann et al., 2017). Gutermann et al. (2017) found that leadership engagement improved follower engagement and job performance. Although this type of leadership is still used in many organizations, transformational leadership is frequently used by nurse leaders, especially in

Magnet®-designated healthcare organizations as it is one of the standards of the American Nurse Credentialing Center. Today's nursing leaders must be able to transform organizations. Nursing leaders must help prepare their organizations for the future, guide team members in embracing change, and influence behaviors, attitudes, and beliefs (Wolters Kluwer, 2017). Transformational leadership was introduced by Burns (1978). It was further developed by Bass and Avolio (1994), who expanded it and identified four concepts: inspirational motivation, intellectual stimulation, individual considerations, and idealized influence (Lappalainen et al., 2020).

The transformational leader is known as a charismatic leader who influences subordinates to meet the goals of the organization. Transformational leaders help subordinates realize their full potential, understand the importance of their tasks, and put the good of the organization above their personal needs (Bolden et al., 2003; George & Jones, 2005). You-De (2013) posits that transactional leadership and transformational leadership can be used by leaders interchangeably. Bass (1985) compared transactional and transformational leadership styles and presented the merits of both, citing transformational leadership as the most effective but adding that at times a transactional leadership style is warranted.

Essential Facts

"Transformational leaders work through empowerment, motivation, consideration, and influence. They listen, affirm, communicate, and exercise a good deal of creativity in how they approach obstacles" (Wolters Kluwer, 2017)

Transformational leadership is a theory in which leaders encourage, inspire, and motivate followers.

This theory is used when an organization needs to be revitalized, is undergoing significant change, or requires a new direction. It is especially vital to today's fast-paced technological industry where innovation and agility can make or break an organization (Flynn, 2019).

The development of a transformational leadership style has been correlated with reduced turnover, improved staff satisfaction, increased care quality and patient satisfaction, and strengthened group commitment to the organization. Leaders who empower their team members help them develop the qualities needed in today's healthcare organizations. According to Berke (2021), transformational leadership is a mindset about being better, which leads to creativity and innovation in the leader and the team. Transformational leaders can easily adapt to new changes and are always seeking to improve outcomes. Transformational leaders are guided by ethics, morals, and integrity and put their values and the values of the company above most others, which inspires team members to do the same.

According to Bass and Bass (2008), these are the hallmarks of transformational leadership that sets it apart from other leadership styles. A transformational leader exemplifies moral standards and serves as a mentor and coach who fosters an ethical work environment. These types of leaders encourage and motivate followers and help them to develop and learn and encourage them to become self-directed (White, 2018).

Kouzes and Posner (2008) developed a model of transformational leadership based on transformational leadership theory. They have been researching and developing their leadership theory for more than 25 years, and based on this research, they have developed the five essential leadership competencies of effective leaders:

1. Model the way.
2. Inspire a share vision.
3. Challenge the process.
4. Enable others to act.
5. Encourage the heart.

Leaders who "model the way" establish principles and standards of excellence for others to follow and create opportunities for others to become successful. Leaders who "inspire a shared vision" believe in their ability to make a difference. They envision the image of the organization and through magnetism enlist others in their dreams. Leaders who "challenge the process" seek to change the status quo. They take risks and set interim goals for small wins as they guide others in achieving larger objectives. Leaders foster collaboration and build spirited teams. They actively involve others. Leaders understand that mutual respect sustains extraordinary efforts. They strive to create an atmosphere of trust and human dignity. They strengthen others, making each person feel capable and powerful. Leaders who "enable others to act" build teams and foster collaboration. They strive to create an atmosphere of human dignity and trust and help others feel capable. Leaders who "encourage the heart" celebrate accomplishments and reward individuals for their contributions and make people feel like heroes (The Leadership Challenge, 2021). Leadership theories have evolved throughout the years, and although transformational leadership has been widely embraced by nursing, theories are always being developed or refined.

LEADERSHIP STYLE

Leadership style is unique, and at times, different styles work better. Authoritative leaders are highly effective in certain situations. "Authoritative leaders mobilize people toward a vision" (Goleman, 2000, p. 80). The clear vision of the leader can motivate others and helps them understand the significance of their contribution (Goleman, 2000). Goleman (2000) describes the authoritative leadership style and how it directs people but offers flexibility in how to achieve the goals. The democratic style of leadership is more collaborative. A democratic leader collaborates with the team to set goals for the future. "This approach is ideal when a leader is himself uncertain about the best direction to take and needs ideas and guidance from able employees" (Goleman, 2000, p. 85). When leaders are striving to motivate others and improve morale, the affiliative style is preferred. Effective leaders of today need to coach and influence individuals instead of coercing them into compliance. The leader can promote acceptance to change when the stakeholders are respected and the programs represent high-quality standards and satisfaction (Green, 2005).

Transformation leadership is considered one of the most effective styles of leadership in healthcare settings. Transformational leadership is the preferred style of Magnet hospitals and has been correlated with increased job satisfaction and decreased turnover in nurses. Nurse managers who promote positive work environments and foster positive attitudes and communication will influence job satisfaction and retention (Lockhart 2015; Moon et al., 2019).

Transformational leadership is correlated with patient safety and outcomes. Leaders play a significant role in promoting a culture of safety (Ree & Wigg, 2019). A study was conducted by Ree and Wigg on the relationship between transformational leadership and patient safety in home care. Several studies emphasize the role of leaders in building a safety culture (Merrill, 2015; Wagner et al., 2018; Wong et al., 2013). McFadden et al. (2009) found that transformational leadership was directly related to patient safety culture and indirectly related to patient safety outcomes through culture and patient safety initiatives, such as education and training of employees and system redesign (Ree & Wigg, 2019, para. 3). Ree (2020) found that transformational leadership and staffing and communication are related to patient-centered care in nursing homes and home care.

Transformational leadership is correlated with a positive work environment, job satisfaction, and patient outcomes. Nursing leaders develop leadership skills that are aligned with those of the transformational leader. Leadership styles may need to be adjusted in specific situations; however, the autocratic and laissez-faire styles are only effective in some situations. McFadden et al. (2015) found that transformational leadership in combination with continuous quality improvement and safety climate improved patient safety outcomes. According to Fischer (2017), a factor in improving patient safety is the development of transformational leadership skills in all nurses.

EMOTIONAL INTELLIGENCE

Emotional intelligence (EQ) is a concept that was popularized by Daniel Goleman in 1995. Although he did not develop the concept, he did write about it extensively. Goleman (1995) expanded on Mayer's and Salovey's four branches of emotional intelligence and described five essential elements of EQ:

1. Emotional self-awareness
2. Self-regulation
3. Motivation
4. Empathy
5. Social skills

EQ is described as the ability to manage one's emotions and the ability to harness those emotions and utilize them for problem-solving. It also includes the ability to help others manage their emotions too (Riggio, 2021). EQ in nurse managers with a master's degree in nursing scored significantly higher in the using emotions branch score than did those with a masters' degree in a related field (Prufeta, 2017). Spano-Szekely et al. (2016) concluded that EQ is a characteristic of transformational leadership in nurse managers which is correlated with patient outcomes. According to Codier and Codier (2017), EQ is related to improved individual and team performance, supports constructive conflict resolution, and improves communication, which is related to patient safety. EQ has many positive benefits. EQ is important for nurse managers and nurses. Nurses with high levels of EQ can manage workloads and handle stress better. It is also related to improved communication and improved patient outcomes (Al-Hamdan et al., 2021).

Emotional skills in nursing are extremely important and benefit patients and colleagues. Nurse managers can help nurses develop their emotional skills by advising them to assess their own strengths and weaknesses and their own reaction to situations (Techniques to Improve Nursing Staff's Emotional Intelligence, 2019). Kutash (2015) concluded that there was a correlation between a nurse's EQ and patient outcomes. However, the relationship was not strong, and further study is warranted. Mansel and Einion (2019) posit that those leaders who possess high levels of EQ are positive role models for their staff. Furthermore, helping staff develop EQ is correlated with quality of care. They conducted a qualitative study and made the following conclusions.

The following key elements appear to be essential to ensuring emotionally intelligent nurse leadership: understanding the concept of EQ in healthcare leadership; recognizing that this will enhance nurse–leadership approaches; placing a high priority on overcoming barriers to effective nurse leadership; committing time and resources to making it happen; ensuring the support of senior management through their demonstration of presence; and visible and emotionally intelligent leadership at all levels of the organizational hierarchy (Mansel & Einion, 2019, p. 1407).

The significance of EQ in nurses and nursing leaders in patient safety and outcomes has been established, and there are ways to develop it. According to Mind Tools (2021), the following strategies can be used to develop EQ:

- Observe how you react to people.
- Look at your work environment.
- Practice humility.
- Self-evaluate.
- Take the EQ quiz.
- Examine how you respond to stressful situations.
- Take responsibility for your actions.

Self-reflection is always a good strategy, and it is important to identify your strengths and weaknesses. EQ is foundational for transformational leaders and can be developed (Butler, 2021). "The value of effective, emotionally intelligent nursing leadership on ensuring safe, quality patient care is unquestionable" (Butler, 2021, para. 25). Butler (2021) described the following skills as essential for emotionally intelligent nurse leaders:

- Self-awareness
- Empathy
- Social skills
- Self-regulation

EQ is a lifelong journey and strategies to improve it should be employed both formally and informally. Workshops, competency evaluations, and self-directed learning can help facilitate the level of EQ.

CRITICAL THINKING AND EMOTIONAL INTELLIGENCE

Critical thinking (CT) goes part and parcel with emotional intelligence and the development of both important skills should begin in the formative years and continue throughout one's life. Zahra and Mansoureh (2015) found that nurses who had a higher level of EQ and awareness tended to have a higher level of CT. Teaching and empowering nurses to attain these skills can improve the quality of nursing care and patient outcomes. CT and EQ are vital skills that should be developed in nursing school. Interestingly, Cheshire et al. (2020) found that EQ scores decreased in baccalaureate nursing students from the beginning to the end of the program. Hasanpour et al. (2018) posit that EQ and CT skills can be learned. Faculty should use active learning and student-centered methods to help students develop these skills, which include the following:

- Team teaching
- Self-learning
- Brainstorming
- Brainstorming
- Concept mapping
- Mind mapping
- Problem-solving,
- Socratic questioning
- Role modeling

Christianson (2020) completed an integrative review of CT and EQ in nursing students that revealed three major themes:

1. EQ and CT are critical for success in nursing education.
2. EQ and CT are interdependent.
3. Nursing education should enhance EQ and CT.

Christianson (2020) concluded that EQ and CT skills and implementing strategies for nursing students throughout their nursing programs deserve thoughtful consideration. Furthermore, nursing programs should consider adding it as an adjunct criterion for admission. Clearly, helping students and nurses improve their EQ skills along with CT skills is important. Michelangelo (2015) completed a meta-analysis and concluded that evidence supports EQ training in nurses and improves CT skills. The author recommended the inclusion of these skills in nursing schools.

SUMMARY

Leaders play a vital role in healthcare organizations and must serve as role models for all members of the healthcare team. Leadership theories have evolved throughout the years, and while there are pros and cons to the theories, transformational leadership is preferred in today's healthcare arena. EQ and CT are necessary skills for nurse leaders who must serve as role models for their nursing team. EQ and CT can be developed and require ongoing development. Both essential skills are correlated with patient outcomes.

VIGNETTE

Joe is a new nurse manager, and his unit has had a sudden increase in patient falls and pressure ulcers. He has been observing the staff and has reprimanded one in front of his peers for not following the correct policy. Was this the proper way to handle the situation? What type of leadership skills do you believe Joe is exhibiting? Do you think he has a high level of EQ? What would you do to help Joe with his leadership? What might be done to improve outcomes?

Discussion Questions

1. Select one leadership theory and provide a summary of the theory and its relevance today.
2. What type of leadership style is preferred in nursing?
3. What is the nurse leader's role throughout the patient care process?
4. How is EQ related to patient outcomes?
5. What is the relationship between CT and EQ?

TIPS FROM THE FIELD

The Emotional Intelligence Work 6 seconds offers 10 tips for developing emotional intelligence:

- Get fluent in the language of emotions
- Name your emotions
- Use the third person when sharing feelings
- Observe without trying to fix
- Feel your emotions in your body
- Bust the myth of bad emotions
- Recognize the recurring patterns
- Notice the buildup before the trigger
- Write down your feelings throughout the day
- Remind yourself that emotions are data

(www.6seconds.org/2018/02/27/emotional-intelligence-tips-awareness)

SPECIAL TOPICS: LEADERSHIP DEVELOPMENT

Developing one's leadership style and skills as a leader is important for all leaders. All your experiences will impact the type of leader you become. Although some leaders are born, most of us need to build on our skills and continue to learn and grow as leaders. In my doctoral dissertation, I focused on the relationship of congruency of leadership support and the value of patient outcomes between nurses and their managers. The primary focus was to examine the relationship of these variables to job satisfaction and turnover in nurses. In my study, I used Kouzes and Posner's Leadership Practice Inventory (LPI, 2002), which measures the five leadership practices described in their model (model the way, inspire a shared vision, challenge the process, enable others to act, encourage the heart; Kouzes & Posner 2007). Kouzes and Posner (2007) have developed two instruments; one is for the leader to use to self-evaluate leadership skills, and the other is for the followers to evaluate their leaders' skills across the five practices. This is a wonderful exercise to use to see how closely aligned you are with the five exemplary practices of a transformational leader.

SUGGESTED CLASSROOM OR UNIT-BASED ASSIGNMENT

Work in small groups. Each student should complete the leadership style quiz at the following URL. Discuss the results and whether you believe this is a true evaluation of your leadership style.

(https://eml.usc.edu/leadership-style-quiz)

RESOURCES

Hannah, S. T., Sumanth, J. J., Lester, P., & Cavarretta, F. (2014). Debunking the false dichotomy of leadership idealism and pragmatism: Critical evaluation and support of newer genre leadership theories. *Journal of Organizational Behavior, 35*(5), 598–621. https://doi-org.libproxy.adelphi.edu/10.1002/job.1931

https://online.ben.edu/programs/msn/resources/five-ways-nursing-leadership-affects-patient-outcomes

Hunt, D. (2014). *The nurse professional: Leveraging your education for transition into practice* (1st ed.). Springer Publishing Company.

Michelangelo, L. (2015). The overall impact of emotional intelligence on nursing students and nursing. *Asia-Pacific Journal of Oncology Nursing*, *2*(2), 118–124. https://doi.org/10.4103/2347-5625.157596

Raghubir, A. E. (2018). Emotional intelligence in professional nursing practice: A concept review using Rodgers's evolutionary analysis approach. *International Journal of Nursing Sciences*, *5*(2), 126–130. https://doi.org/10.1016/j.ijnss.2018.03.004

REFERENCES

Al-Hamdan, Z. M., Alyahia, M., Al-Maaitah, R., Alhamdan, M., Faouri, I., Al-Smadi, A. M., & Bawadi, H. (2021). The relationship between emotional intelligence and nurse–nurse collaboration. *Journal of Nursing Scholarship*, *53*(5), 615–622. https://doi.org/10.1111/jnu.12687

Bass, B. (1985). *Leadership and performance beyond expectations.* New York: Free Press.

Bass, B. M., & Avolio, B. J. (1994). *Improving organizational effectiveness through transformational leadership.* Thousand Oaks, CA: Sage Publications.

Bass, B. M., & Bass, R. (2008). *Handbook of leadership: Theory, research, and application.* Free Press.

Benmira, S., & Agboola, M. (2021). Evolution of leadership theory. *BMJ Leader*, *5*, 3–5.

Bennis, W. G. (2009). *On becoming a leader.* Basic Books.

Berke, A. (2021). *Transformational leadership.* https://www.workpatterns.com/articles/transformational-leadership

Bolden, R., Gosling, J., Marturano, A., & Dennison, P. (2003). *A review of leadership theory and competency frameworks.* Centre for Leadership Studies, http://www.leadersh studies.com/ documents/mgmtstandards.pdf

Buchanan, D. A., & Huczynski, A. (2017). *Organizational behaviour.* (9th ed.). Pearson Education Limited.

Burns, J. M. (1978). *Leadership.* New York: Harper & Row.

Butler, J. (2021). Emotional intelligence in nursing leadership. *Australian Nursing & Midwifery Journal, 27*(5), 18.

Cheshire, M. H., Strickland, H. P., & Ewell, P. J. (2020). Measured emotional intelligence in baccalaureate nursing education: A longitudinal study. *Nursing Education Perspectives, 41*(2), 103–105. https://doi.org/10.1097/01.NEP.0000000000000476

Christianson, K. L. (2020).Emotional intelligence and critical thinking in nursing students: Integrative review of literature. *Nurse Educator, 45*(6), E62–E65. https://doi.org/10.1097/NNE.0000000000000801

Codier, E., & Codier, D. D. (2017). Could emotional intelligence make patients safer? *American Journal of Nursing, 117*(7), 58–62. https://doi.org/10.1097/01.NAJ.0000520946.39224.db

Derue, S. D., Nahrgang, J. D., Wellman, N., & Humphrey, S. E. (2011). Trait and behavioral theories of leadership: An integration and meta-analytic test of their relative validity. *Personnel Psychology, 64*(1), 7–52. https://doi.org/10.1111/j.1744-6570.2010.01201.x

Fiedler, F. E. (1967). *A theory of leadership effectiveness.* NewYork: McGraw-Hill.

Fischer, S. A. (2017). Developing nurses' transformational leadership skills. *Nursing Standard, 31*(51), 54. http://dx.doi.org/10.7748/ns.2017.e10857

Fielder, F., & Chemers, M. (1974). *Leadership and effective management.* Glenville, IL: Scott Foresman and Co.

Flynn, S. I. (2019). *Transformational and transactional leadership.* Great Neck Publishing.

George, J., & Jones, G. (2005). *Understanding and managing organizational behavior* (4th ed.). Pearson-Prentice Hall.

Goleman, D. (1995). *Emotional intelligence.* Bantam Books.

Goleman, D. (2000). *Leadership that gets results.* Harvard Business Review.

Green, R. (2005). *Practicing the art of leadership* (2nd ed.). Upper Saddle River, NJ: Pearson-Prentice Hall.

Gutermann, D., Lehmann, W. N., Boer, D., Born, M., & Voelpel, S. C. (2017). How leaders affect followers' work engagement and performance: Integrating leader–member exchange and crossover theory. *British Journal of Management, 28*(2), 299–314. https://doi-org.libproxy.adelphi.edu/10.1111/1467-8551.12214

Hasanpour, M., Bagheri, M., & Ghaedi Heidari, F. (2018). The relationship between emotional intelligence and critical thinking skills in Iranian nursing students. *Medical Journal of the Islamic Republic of Iran, 32*, 40. https://doi.org/10.14196/mjiri.32.40

Hunt, D. (2012). *Nurses' and supervisors' value congruence, leadership support and patient outcomes and the effect on job satisfaction and intent to leave (Order No. 3504805).* Dissertations & Theses, Adelphi University; ProQuest Central; ProQuest Dissertations & Theses Global. (1000476786). http://libproxy.adelphi.edu/login?url=https://www.proquest.com/dissertations-theses/nurses-supervisors-value-congruence-leadership/docview/1000476786/se-2

Kouzes, J., & Posner, B. (2002). *The leadership practices inventory, (LPI).* http://www.leadershipchallenge.com

Kouzes, J., & Posner, B. (2007). *The leadership practices inventory, (LPI).* http://www.leadershipchallenge.com

Kouzes, J., & Posner, B. (2008). *The leadership challenge* (4th ed.). Jossey Bass.

Kouzes, J., & Posner, B. (2010). *The leadership practices inventory, (LPI).* http://www.leadershipchallenge.com

Kutash, M. (2015). *The relationship between nurses' emotional intelligence and patient outcomes.* ProQuest Dissertations Publishing.

Lappalainen, M., Härkänen, M., & Kvist, T. (2020). The relationship between nurse manager's transformational leadership style and medication safety. *Scandinavian Journal of Caring Sciences, 34*(2), 357–369. https://doi-org.libproxy.adelphi.edu/10.1111/scs.12737

The Leadership Challenge. (2021). *Discover The Five Practices of Exemplary Leadership.* https://www.leadershipchallenge.com/Research/Five-Practices.aspx

Lockhart, L. (2015). Find your inner transformational leader. *Nursing Made Incredibly Easy, 13*(4), 55. https://doi.org/10.1097/01.NME.0000465776.13006.04

Mansel, B., & Einion, A. (2019). "It's the relationship you develop with them": Emotional intelligence in nurse leadership. A qualitative study. *British Journal of Nursing, 28*(21), 1400–1408. https://doi-org.libproxy.adelphi.edu/10.12968/bjon.2019.28.21.1400

McFadden, K. L., Henagan, S. C., & Gowen, C. R. (2009). The patient safety chain: Transformational leadership's effect on patient safety culture, initiatives, and outcomes. *Journal of Operations Management, 27*(5), 390–404. https://doi.org/10.1016/j.jom.2009.01.001

McFadden, K. L., Stock, G. N., & Gowen, C. R. (2015). Leadership, safety climate, and continuous quality improvement. *Health Care Management Review, 40*(1), 24–34. https://doi.org/10.1097/hmr.0000000000000006

Merrill, K. C. (2015). Leadership style and patient safety: Implications for nurse managers. *Journal of Nursing Administration, 45*(6), 319–324. https://doi.org/10.1097/NNA.0000000000000207

Michelangelo, L. (2015). The overall impact of emotional intelligence on nursing students and nursing. *Asia-Pacific Journal of Oncology Nursing, 2*(2), 118–124. https://doi.org/10.4103/2347-5625.157596

Mind Tools. (2021). *Emotional intelligence: Developing strong people skills.* https://www.mindtools.com/pages/article/newCDV_59.htm

Moon, S. E., Van Dam, P. J., & Kitsos, A. (2019). Measuring transformational leadership in establishing nursing care excellence. *Healthcare, 7*(4), 132. https://doi.org/10.3390/healthcare7040132

Prufeta, P. (2017). Emotional intelligence of nurse managers: An exploratory study. *Journal of Nursing Administration, 47*(3), 134–139. https://doi.org/10.1097/NNA.0000000000000455

Ree, E. (2020). What is the role of transformational leadership, work environment and patient safety culture for person-centred care? A cross-sectional study in Norwegian nursing homes and home care services. *Nursing Open*, *7*(6), 1988–1996. http://dx.doi.org/10.1002/nop2.592

Ree, E., & Wiig, S. (2019). Linking transformational leadership, patient safety culture and work engagement in home care services. *Nursing Open*, *7*(1), 256–264. https://doi.org/10.1002/nop2.386

Riggio, R. (2021, September 22). *The Truth About Emotional Intelligence*. Psychology Today. https://www.psychologytoday.com/us/blog/cutting-edge-leadership/202109/the-truth-about-emotional-intelligence

Spano-Szekely, L., Quinn Griffin, M. T., Clavelle, J., & Fitzpatrick, J. J. (2016). Emotional intelligence and transformational leadership in nurse managers. *Journal of Nursing Administration*, *46*(2), 101–108. https://doi.org/10.1097/NNA.0000000000000303

Techniques to Improve Nursing Staff's Emotional Intelligence. (2019). Same – Day Surgery, *43*(11) http://libproxy.adelphi.edu/login?url=https://www.proquest.com/trade-journals/techniques-improve-nursing-staff-s-emotional/docview/2304833388/se-2?accountid=8204

Vecchio, R. P., Justin, J. E., & Pearce, C. L. (2008). The utility of transactional and transformational leadership for predicting performance and satisfaction within a path-goal theory framework. *Journal of Occupational & Organizational Psychology*, *81*(1), 71–82. https://doi-org.libproxy.adelphi.edu/10.1348/096317907X202482

Wagner, A., Hammer, A., Manser, T., Martus, P., Sturm, H., & Rieger, M. (2018). Do occupational and patient safety culture in hospitals share predictors in the field of psychosocial working conditions? Findings from a cross-sectional study in German university hospitals. *International Journal of Environmental Research and Public Health*, *15*(10), 2131. https://doi.org/10.3390/ijerph15102131

White, S. K. (2018). *What is transformational leadership?* https://www.cio.com/article/3257184/what-is-transformational-leadership-a-model-for-motivating-innovation.html

Wolters Kluwer. (2017). *At the core of Magnet: Transformational leadership.* https://www.wolterskluwer.com/en/expert-insights/at-the-core-of-magnet-transformational-leadership

Wong, C. A., Cummings, G. G., & Ducharme, L. (2013). The relationship between nursing leadership and patient outcomes: A systematic review update. *Journal of Nursing Management*, *21*(5), 709–724. https://doi.org/10.1111/jonm.12116

You-De, D., You-Yu, D., Kuan-Yang, C., & Hui-Chun, W. (2013). Transformational vs transactional leadership: Which is better? A study on employees of international tourist hotels in Taipei City. *International Journal of Contemporary Hospitality Management*, *25*(5), 760–778. http://dx.doi.org/10.1108/IJCHM-Dec-2011-0223

Yukl, G. (1971). Toward a behavioral theory of leadership. *Organizational Behavior and Human Performance*, *6*(4), 414–440. https://doi.org/10.1016/0030-5073(71)90026-2”>https://doi.org/10.1016/0030-5073(71)90026-2; https://www.sciencedirect.com/science/article/pii/0030507371900262

Zahra, M., & Mansoureh N. (2015). Critical thinking in nurses: Predictive role of emotional intelligence. *Hayāt*, *20*(4), 77–88.

8

A Holistic Approach for Nurses: Putting the Pieces Together for Safe, Effective Care

Caring is the Essence of Nursing.

—Jean Watson

The preceding chapters discussed various issues surrounding patient safety and ways to improve patient outcomes. This final chapter provides a holistic perspective and highlights ways to integrate the information so you can identify best practices and incorporate them into your approach to patient safety, quality of care, and patient outcomes.

In this chapter, you will learn:

1. Holistic/Integrative practices and patient outcomes
2. Nursing process and Patient Outcomes
3. Improving Patient Safety
4. Cultural beliefs and patient outcomes
5. Putting the pieces together

Taking a holistic approach to patient safety doesn't mean applying all strategies at the same time; it means intentionally thinking about each patient as an individual and, with the goal to do no harm, providing evidenced-based quality of care and promoting positive patient outcomes. Approaching this from the lens of the nursing process can help guide you in the journey to becoming a safer healthcare provider.

ASSESSMENT OF PROBLEM

Assessing patients, and indeed any problem, is always the first step. In Chapter 1, you read about the major issues in patient safety and adverse events. It is important to understand the perils and pitfalls so you know what to avoid and can plan how to avoid being part of the problem versus the solution. There are all types of errors, and while many are multidisciplinary, and due to a breakdown in process or poorly written policies and procedures, there are some that relate specifically to the discipline. "Nursing-sensitive indicators are the criteria for changes in health status that nursing care can directly affect" (Joint Commission International, 2014; Nakrem et al., 2009, as cited in Oner et al., 2020, p. 1006). These nursing-sensitive indicators include medication errors, patient falls, pressure ulcers, hospital-acquired infections, mortality, failure to rescue, length of stay, nurse satisfaction, and patient satisfaction (Oner et al., 2020). Knowing the magnitude of the problem and how this relates to your scope of practice is key. To examine institution-specific problems, you can include your quality improvement team. You can also search national databases and The Joint Commission for the high-risk areas.

The next step is to examine the root causes of these adverse events. In Chapter 2, the primary causes were poor communication, causes and types of medication errors, misuse of technology, poorly conceived processes and execution, and workload issues. Are there other issues and causes? Assessing the various types of causes can help you identify ways to avoid them. This requires a significant amount of self-reflection on your knowledge, skills, and attitudes. What is your knowledge gap? How will you obtain the knowledge that you need? What skills do you need to improve? Are you fully committed to promoting positive patient outcomes? Have you had "near misses," or have you made an error? If so, how did it make you feel? What caused the error? What changes, if any, were made to policy and procedures? What changes did you make to help avoid another error? Are you a role model for others? Do you believe you value patient outcomes? Do you believe your nurse manager values patient outcomes? You can both use the Value of Patient Outcomes Scale included at the end of this chapter and compare the results.

PLANNING AND INTERVENTIONS

The plan for becoming a safe practitioner requires short- and long-term planning. There are many ways to become a safer practitioner, educate yourself and students, or facilitate this in team members. Healthcare is in a state of constant flux and requires a commitment to lifelong learning. Education should be general and then specific and competency-based to the type of unit and patients served. Quality improvement must be done on a continual basis. Orientation and professional development and evaluation of performance and evaluation are vital components.

Theory-informed practice requires the integration of a theory into your planning and interventions. For example, Watson's Caring Theory can influence all spheres of care. Redlands Community hospital uses Jean Watson's theory to guide its nursing care and promote positive patient outcomes. "At Redlands Community Hospital, nursing has embraced the theory of Jean Watson's Caring Science. Caring Science helps us to embrace the positive energy that flows from an integrated mind, body and spirit and is mutually rewarding to both the patient and the nurse. By actively engaging in caring through authentic presence and intentionality, the nurse is able to optimize her patient's ability to heal from within" (Redlands Community Hospital, 2021, para. 1). Jean Watson's theory of caring and the 10 carative factors have been used as the theoretical and philosophical underpinnings of many academic and healthcare institutions. There are other theories that can be used individually or in combination with other theories.

The nursing process requires the nurse to utilize critical thinking, reasoning, and logic throughout the assessment, planning, interventions, and evaluation. Prioritization and delegation are required to ensure the interventions are done to promote positive patient outcomes.

EVALUATION

Evaluation is an important step in the nursing process and must be done on a continual basis. This also requires critical thinking, reasoning, and logic as each intervention is evaluated for its effectiveness. The planning process should list the patient outcomes you will be measuring to evaluate the effectiveness of the various interventions. If the interventions are not effective the plan would be revised. The goal is to have zero adverse events and high levels of compliance; however, there are some adverse events, such as pressure ulcers that are not preventable so the plan should be realistic with achievable goals.

Being mindful of patient safety and understanding the significant role you play in creating a safe environment for patients, families, and staff are keys to improving patient outcomes. Having the knowledge, skills, and attitudes in addition to technology and other tools available will help you promote a culture of safety.

Essential Facts

The causal relationship between nurse-to-patient ratios and patient outcomes likely is accounted for by both increased workload and stress, and the risk of burnout for nurses. The high-intensity nature of nurses' work means that nurses themselves are at risk of committing errors while providing routine care (Malliaris et al., 2021).

CULTURE AND PATIENT SAFETY

"Culture and Patient Outcomes Culture can be defined as the "personal identification, language, thoughts, communications, actions, customs, beliefs, values, and institutions that are often specific to ethnic, racial, religious, geographic, or social groups" (Agency for Healthcare Research and Quality [AHRQ], 2019, para. 1). All healthcare institutions are expected to have a culture of safety, and they are required to provide education on cultural concepts and include it as part of the annual competency development and assessment of all staff. Failure to address culture, health literacy, and language barriers have all been correlated with adverse events. Cultural competence can improve patient engagement and patient outcomes (AHRQ, 2019). The current focus has shifted away from cultural competency and is now focused on cultural humility as one can never truly be culturally competent as there are so many different cultures and nuances within cultures:

"The Center for Health Equity Advancement (CHEA) describes cultural humility as the ongoing process of developing a set of skills to approach any individual from any culture at any time. Cultural humility focuses on lifelong learning, self-reflection, removing power differentials (such as provider and patient), and demonstrating equal respect for different beliefs and points of view" (Shuster, 2021).

Cultural humility involves openness to cultural individuals and groups. When perceptions of organizational cultural humility increase, there is a higher level of perceptions of patient safety (Handtke et al., 2019; Hook et al., 2016).

Essential Facts

"Cultural humility is a lifelong process of self-reflection which is also defined by that individual. It allows an individual to be open to other people's identities, which is core to the nursing standard of providing holistic care" (Hughes et al., 2020, p. 28).

Promoting and educating about cultural humility in academia and healthcare settings can be done in a variety of ways. In academic programs, the content should be threaded throughout the curriculum. In healthcare settings, it should be included in orientation and annual education and competency programs. Simulation is an excellent way to teach nurses and other healthcare practitioners about cultural humility and Immersion experiences can also be beneficial when feasible. Journaling and service-learning can also be used to develop cultural humility (Hughes et al., 2020).

THE FUTURE OF HEALTHCARE AND ARTIFICIAL INTELLIGENCE

Artificial intelligence will continue to be used to improve patient outcomes. "Artificial intelligence (AI) provides opportunities to identify the health risks of patients and thus influence patient safety outcomes" (Choudhury & Asan, 2020). A systematic review was completed by Choudhury and Asan (2020), and they concluded that AI-enabled decision support systems can improve patient safety in the areas of drug management, patient stratification, and error detection. However, future research is required to ensure AI is implemented correctly and to understand how well it can predict patient safety and outcomes.

According to Bates et al. (2021) AI can be used to improve patient safety and can be used in various settings, inpatient, outpatient, and home and community settings. Technology and AI can be used in various ways to identify high-risk patients, improve communication, and decrease preventable harms. LABline (2021) discussed the benefits of AI, which include accuracy of diagnosing, improved research on health and medications, assistance with clinical care, and support for diverse public health initiatives. However, the recommendations of the World Health Organization also caution against overestimating the benefits and unethical behaviors in data collection and risks to patient data and cybersecurity.

AI is still being developed and will continue to have risks and benefits. Research must continue to identify best practices in the use of AI and other technologies that will continue to improve patient outcomes.

SUMMARY

This chapter provided a strategy for using the nursing process to put the pieces together and develop short- and long-range goals for improving patient outcomes. An exemplar from a hospital that has used Jean Watson's caring theory was also highlighted. The relationship between cultural humility and patient safety was discussed, and the pros and cons of artificial intelligence (AI) in the healthcare setting.

VIGNETTE

Mr. Goodman, RN, is the nurse manager on a surgical intensive care unit. During the past 3 months, there has been an increase in falls and medication errors. How can Mr. Goodman use the nursing process to create a short- and long-range plan to address these serious issues? Who should be included in the plan? What teaching pedagogies/strategies can be utilized? The staff believe the errors are related to high patient-to-nurse ratios, which have been impacted by the COVID-19 pandemic. However, the errors occur even on days when there are low patient-to-nurse ratios. What types of data does he need? What components would be important to include in the plan? What resources are required? How will he evaluate the effectiveness of the plan? What should be done if the plan has been successful? What should be done if the plan has not been successful?

Discussion Questions

1. What are the steps of the nursing process?
2. What is meant by theory-informed practice?
3. Describe cultural humility and how it is correlated with patient outcomes?
4. How is AI currently being used in healthcare settings?
5. List two resources you can use to increase your knowledge of patient safety.

TIPS FROM THE FIELD: SIMULATION AND MEDICATION SAFETY

Healthcare simulation provides an opportunity to teach healthcare practitioners about medication safety (Baily, 2020). "The purpose of the ISMP Targeted Medication Safety Best Practices for Hospitals is to identify, inspire, and mobilize widespread, national adoption of consensus-based Best Practices for specific medication safety issues that continue to cause fatal and harmful errors in patients, despite repeated warnings in ISMP publications" (Baily, 2020, para. 6).

Educators can use the information from the following website, along with the Institute for Safe Medication Practice worksheet, to create targeted simulation experiences.

www.healthysimulation.com/23457/institute-for-safe-medication-practices-healthcare-simulation/?fbclid=IwAR2BcBa9MDCgvJg333Ff9wPZ4alGj_66YMZ0LSTOFqPtcvkBOLg8N6TiAfc

You must sign up for a free account to access the tools and worksheets at the following website:

www.ismp.org/resources/worksheet-ismp-targeted-medication-safety-best-practices-hospitals

SPECIAL TOPICS: THE VALUE OF PATIENT OUTCOMES SCALE

The Value of Patient Outcomes Scale (Hunt, 2011) compares the nurse's value of patient outcomes to his/her supervisor's value of patient outcomes. There are eight questions with a Likert scale that ranges from SA = *Strongly Agree* to SD = *Strongly Disagree*. Possible scores range from 8 to 32 with the higher scores indicating a higher value of patient outcomes. This instrument was developed based on current research findings that describe the common attitudes and beliefs that nurses would identify related to patient quality of care and patient outcomes. For example, the literature suggests that patient outcomes include adverse outcomes, nosocomial infections, decreased length of stay, falls, pressure ulcers, and failure to rescue (AHRC, 2007; Needleman et al., 2002; TJC, 2010). Content and face validity were established by a panel of five experts in the field of quality and patient outcomes (Hunt, 2011). (See Appendices 1 and 2.)

SUGGESTED CLASSROOM OR UNIT-BASED ASSIGNMENT

Have students or staff work in small groups to create a short- and long-range plan for promoting positive patient outcomes.

- What issue will be addressed?
- What is the evidence for the policy and procedure related to the treatment or skill?
- How will you implement the updated protocol or policy/procedure?
- What resources are needed?
- How will you evaluate it?

CASE EXEMPLAR 8.1: QUALITY MANAGEMENT IN TELEPHONE TRIAGE

Christine Rovinski-Wagner

Safety is the highest quality outcome nurses provide to patients. For instance, a newly licensed nurse identifies an incorrect surgical site mark for a patient scheduled for a lumbar puncture in interventional radiology. The nurse was expecting a mark in the lumbar region but finds the site mark on the patient's shoulder. The nurse asks a clinical nurse leader (CNL) to cross-check the assessment. The CNL validates the error, and the physician returns to re-mark the patient in the appropriate lumbar region before the patient is transferred to the procedure room. The nurse's use of structure (having the resource of a clinical nurse leader) and process (using a standardized preprocedural checklist and seeking the assistance of a more experienced nurse) prevented an outcome of potential harm to the patient. Examples of how a nurse can provide safe high-quality nursing in clinic or inpatient health care settings are abundant and obvious. The nurse and the patient are visible to each other. Less obvious, but just as abundant, are the ways telephone triage nurses, in the growing arena of clinical call centers, can demonstrate levels of individual performance that effectively use those healthcare systems to minimize the risk of harm to the patient.

Two measurements for quality management in telephone triage are how quickly a nurse answers incoming calls and the length of time a nurse spends on these calls. The length of time a nurse spends on a telephone call impacts how quickly a nurse is able to answer other calls. These measures, as well as how many calls a nurse answers, are also used as part of a nurse's performance evaluation.

After answering the telephone, the nurse utilizes an evidence-based algorithm, referred to as a decision support tool, to assess the patient's symptoms and determine the recommendation for follow-up care. This recommendation is given to the patient. It is the patient's decision to follow the recommendation or not. The patient's agreement to follow a recommendation is documented and that data are also measured for quality management and performance evaluation.

The telephone triage nurse's use of two elements of shared decision-making, communication of risk in following or not following recommendations and clarifying patient values that influence preferences in obtaining healthcare, is essential for the achievement of safe high-quality outcomes. These both take time. It is the nurse's decision to take the time or not.

Patient Review

A patient called the telephone triage nurse expressing concern about higher than usual blood pressure readings. The patient reported that after taking his blood pressure medications blood pressure was lower and the headache he had experienced was gone. The patient wondered if he should see a doctor sooner than the scheduled appointment with his surgeon. When the nurse asked why he was seeing a surgeon, the patient replied he had a hernia repaired about 4 weeks earlier and that it was just to make sure the surgery fixed the problem. The nurse asked if the patient had noticed anything else different in his health recently. The patient replied he had a quick stab of chest pain several days ago and since then was experiencing some shortness of breath during activity but that was okay because he didn't get out of his chair much during the day.

At this point, the telephone triage nurse asked the patient to stay on the phone and walk around the room. The nurse quickly detected respiratory distress: shortness of breath, audible tachypnea, coughing, and the patient saying, "I am out of breath." The nurse was simultaneously documenting in the decision support tool, with the algorithm disposition recommending emergent care. The telephone triage nurse advised immediate evaluation at a hospital via 911. The patient hesitated to say he would "catch his breath" after sitting still for a few minutes. In response, the nurse told the patient that sometimes inactivity after a surgery could cause blood clots to travel around the body and that his symptoms were consistent with that serious occurrence. The patient kept saying that he didn't want to bother anyone and that "other people are sicker than me." He finally agreed to a 911 evaluation and transfer to a local hospital. A supervising nurse in the clinical call center contacted 911, while the telephone triage nurse kept the patient on the telephone line, framing his need for emergent health care as important as anyone else he might identify as needing it more than he did. When the emergency responders arrived, the telephone triage nurse provided a Situation–Background–Assessment–Recommendation handoff to them. Subsequently, the patient was admitted to the hospital with a pulmonary embolism.

The telephone triage nurse could have reassured the patient about normal blood pressure values, provided positive reinforcement for taking medications, and ended the triage call. The quality performance measurements of speed to answer and length of call would have met predetermined targets. Instead, the nurse did not meet the targets by making the right choice to focus on and address the patient's needs. The nurse demonstrated an exemplary level of individual nursing practice by carefully obtaining a detailed history from the patient about his health concerns, skillfully evaluating the patient's physical status within the constraints of the practice setting, fully triaging the patient's health issue, artfully addressing the patient's preferences regarding seeking healthcare services, and effectively using the call center structure to facilitate the patient's transfer to the most appropriate healthcare setting for his condition. The nurse, without seeing or being in the same room as the patient, ensured the safest possible outcome.

RESOURCES

Cultural Respect.nih.gov. https://www.nih.gov/institutes-nih/nih-office-director/office-communications-public-liaison/clear-communication/cultural-respect

https://inclusion.uoregon.edu/trainings-and-other-activities-and-strategies-develop-cultural-humility

www.ismp.org/resources/just-culture-medication-error-prevention-and-second-victim-support-better-prescription

www.ismp.org/resources/white-paper-case-medication-safety-officers-mso

www.ismp.org/system/files/resources/2020-03/2020-2021_ISMP_Targeted_Medication_Safety_Best_Practices_Worksheet_3.pdf

REFERENCES

Agency for Health Care Research and Quality. (2007). *2007 National Healthcare Quality & Disparities Reports*. https://www.ahrq.gov/research/findings/nhqrdr/index.html

Agency for Healthcare Research and Quality. (2019). *Cultural competence and patient safety*. https://psnet.ahrq.gov/perspective/cultural-competence-and-patient-safety

Baily, K. (2020, March 20). *Institute for Safe Medication Practices worksheet useful for healthcare simulation programs*. HealthySimulation.Com. https://www.healthysimulation.com/23457/institute-for-safe-medication-practices-healthcare-simulation/

Bates, D. W., Levine, D., Syrowatka, A., Kuznetsova, M., Craig, A. R., Rui, A., Jackson, G. P., & Rhee, K. (2021). The potential of artificial intelligence to improve patient safety: A scoping review. *NPJ Digital Medicine*, *4*, 54. https://doi.org/10.1038/s41746-021-00423-6

Choudhury, A., & Asan, O. (2020). Role of artificial intelligence in patient safety outcomes: Systematic literature review. *JMIR Medical Informatics*, *8*(7), e18599. https://doi.org/10.2196/18599

Handtke, O., Schilgen, B., & Mosko, M. (2019). Culturally competent healthcare – A scoping review of strategies implemented in healthcare organizations and a model of culturally competent healthcare provision. *PLoS One*. https://doi.org/10.1371/journal.pone.0219971

Hook, J. N., Boan, D., Davis, D. E., Aten, J. D., Ruiz, J. M., & Maryon, T. (2016). Cultural humility and hospital safety culture. *Journal of Clinical Psychology in Medical Settings*, *23*(4), 402–409. doi:10.1007/s10880-016-9471-x

Hughes, V., Delva, S., Nkimbeng, M., Spaulding, E., Turkson-Ocran, R.-A., Cudjoe, J., Ford, A., Rushton, C., D'Aoust, R., & Han, H.-R. (2020). Not missing the opportunity: Strategies to promote cultural humility among future nursing faculty. *Journal of Professional Nursing*, *36*(1), 28–33. https://doi.org/10.1016/j.profnurs.2019.06.005; https://www.sciencedirect.com/science/article/pii/S8755722319300869)

Hunt, D. (2011). Nurses' and supervisors' value congruence, leadership support, and patient outcomes and the effect on job satisfaction and intent to leave. Thesis (Ph. D.)–Adelphi University, 2011. Print.

LABline. (2021, December 7). *Machine learning may help identify people at risk of thoracic aortic aneurysm*. Medical Laboratory Observer. https://www.mlo-online.com/information-technology/artificial-intelligence/article/21249271/machine-learning-may-help-identify-people-at-risk-of-thoracic-aortic-aneurysm

Malliaris, A., Phillips, J., & Bakerjian, D. (2021). *Nursing and patient safety*. https://psnet.ahrq.gov/primer/nursing-and-patient-safety

Needleman, J., Buerhaus, P., Mattke, S., Stewart, M., & Zelevinsky, K. (2002). Nurse-staffing levels and the quality of care in hospitals. *New England Journal of Medicine*, *346*(22), 1715–1722. https://doi.org/10.1056/nejmsa012247

Oner, B., Zengul, F. D., Oner, N., Ivankova, N. V., Karadag, A., & Patrician, P. A. (2021). Nursing-sensitive indicators for nursing care: A systematic review (1997–2017). *Open Access*. https://doi.org/10.1002/nop2.654

Redlands Community Hospital. (2021). *Jean Watson's Theory of Human Caring.* https://www.redlandshospital.org/nursing-excellence/jean-watsons-theory-of-human-caring/

Shuster, D. (2020). *Honing cultural humility skills can improve health care as a whole.* https://www.pennmedicine.org/news/news-blog/2021/may/honing-cultural-humility-skills-can-improve-health-care-as-a-whole

The Joint Commission (TJC). (2010). *Health care at the crossroads: Strategies for addressing the evolving nursing crisis.* Retrieved from www.iointcommission.org

Appendix 1: Nurse's Value of Patient Outcomes Scale (Nurse)

Deborah A. Hunt
@Hunt 2010

Directions: For each item below, circle the appropriate response.

Response Key: SA = Strongly Agree
A = Agree
D = Disagree
SD = Strongly Disagree

There is no right or wrong answers to these questions.

(Examples of adverse patient outcomes: falls, pressure ulcers, infections, medication errors)

I use patient outcomes in conversations about patients.	SA A D SD
I value bedside care as much as I value patient outcomes.	SA A D SD
My immediate supervisor values patient outcomes just as much as I do.	SA A D SD

Patient satisfaction is more important than patient outcomes.	SA A D SD
I voluntarily participate in a program that tracks required patient outcomes initiated by hospital administration.	SA A D SD
Patient outcomes are important, but they are not my responsibility.	SA A D SD
My colleagues do not value patient outcomes as much as I do.	SA A D SD
Hospital Administration values patient outcomes more than staffing ratios.	SA A D SD

Scoring: For positive items SA = 4; A = 3; D=2; SD = 1.

For negative items SA = 1; A = 2; D= 3; and SD = 4

Appendix 2: Nurse's Value of Patient Outcomes Scale (Supervisor)

Deborah A. Hunt
@Hunt 2010

Directions: For each item below, circle the appropriate response.

Response Key: SA = Strongly Agree
A = Agree
D = Disagree
SD = Strongly Disagree

There is no right or wrong answers to these questions.

(Examples of adverse patient outcomes: falls, pressure ulcers, infections, medication errors)

I use patient outcomes in conversations about patients.	SA A D SD
I value bedside care as much as I value patient outcomes.	SA A D SD

My staff nurses value patient outcomes just as much as I do.	SA A D SD
Patient satisfaction is more important than patient outcomes.	SA A D SD
I voluntarily participate in a program that tracks required patient outcomes initiated by hospital administration.	SA A D SD
Patient outcomes are important, but they are not my responsibility.	SA A D SD
My staff nurses do not value patient outcomes as much as I do.	SA A D SD
Hospital Administration values patient outcomes more than staffing ratios.	SA A D SD

Scoring: For positive items SA = 4; A = 3; D=2; SD = 1.

For negative items SA = 1; A = 2; D= 3; and SD = 4

Index

www.ingramcontent.com/pod-product-compliance
Ingram Content Group UK Ltd.
Pitfield, Milton Keynes, MK11 3LW, UK
UKHW021353110926
15107UKWH00004B/10

9 780826 184559